The Electromyographer's Handbook

The Electromyographer's Handbook

Lowery Lee Thompson, M.D.
Mercy Medical Center, Nampa, Idaho; Formerly Senior Resident in Neurology, University of Utah College of Medicine, Salt Lake City, Utah

Little, Brown and Company   Boston

Published November 1981

Copyright © 1981 by Lowery Lee Thompson

First Edition

All rights reserved. No part of this book may be reproduced in any form or by any electronic or mechanical means, including information storage and retrieval systems, without permission in writing from the publisher, except by a reviewer who may quote brief passages in a review.

Library of Congress Catalog Card No. 81-83244

ISBN 0-316-84185-4

Printed in the United States of America

HAL

To my wife Barbara, who assisted in every phase of production,
and to my daughter Amy

Contents

Preface	ix
1 Introduction to Nerve Conduction Studies	1
2 Brachial Plexus (*Motor Studies*)	13
3 Ulnar Nerve (*Motor and Sensory Studies*)	19
4 Median Nerve (*Motor and Sensory Studies*)	27
5 Radial Nerve (*Motor and Sensory Studies*)	35
6 Musculocutaneous Nerve (*Sensory Studies*)	43
7 Sciatic Nerve (*Motor Studies*)	47
8 Peroneal Nerve (*Motor Studies*)	53
9 Superficial Peroneal Nerve (*Sensory Studies*)	59
10 Tibial Nerve (*Motor Studies*)	63
11 Sural Nerve (*Sensory Studies*)	67
12 Femoral Nerve (*Motor Studies*)	71
13 Saphenous Nerve (*Sensory Studies*)	77
14 Facial Nerve Stimulation (*Motor Studies*)	81
15 The F-Wave	87
16 The H-Reflex	91
17 Slow Repetitive Supramaximal Stimulation of a Motor Nerve	95
18 The EMG Examination	101

Appendixes

I Amplitudes of EMAPs Recorded from Selected Muscles	131
II Durations of EMAPs Recorded by Stimulation of Selected Nerves	132
III The EMG Report Form	133
IV Normal Conduction Velocities and Distal Latencies	134
V The Innervation of Commonly Studied Muscles by Named Nerves and Spinal Segments	136
VI The Major Motor Distributions of Commonly Studied Nerves	138
VII Myotomes of the Upper and Lower Extremities	139
VIII The EMG Examination: Characteristics of Spontaneous and Exertional Activity	141
IX Motor Points of Commonly Studied Muscles	143
Index	151

Preface

The primary purpose of this handbook is to help trainees in electroneuromyography achieve the basic competence in standard procedures necessary for the development of more sophisticated skill in electrodiagnosis. By providing exact information about electrode placement and expected values in a single source, it bridges the gap between the excellent comprehensive textbooks in this field and the specific journal articles that describe each individual technique.

Students at each level, as well as physicians, physical therapists, and technicians who work in an EMG laboratory, should find it a handy reference, especially for those procedures not done on a daily basis. The first seventeen chapters are concerned with techniques of motor and sensory nerve stimulation. Each discussion reviews the relevant anatomy, lists applications, describes the technique, and provides a referenced table of normal values. Every technique is described step by step, and each step is illustrated with drawings and photographs.

The final chapter, on the EMG examination, provides a general introduction to the topic and information about the usual normal and abnormal findings. The concept of recruitment and single motor unit control is discussed in detail, for the correct interpretation of the so-called interference pattern is as difficult as it is important. The appendixes provide summary information in a convenient tabular form.

Specific information is taken from references from 1948 to 1980. Some of the older information is particularly useful because it is not readily available in detail in other current textbooks—for example, duration of motor unit action potentials by muscle and age.

The Electromyographer's Handbook will have met its goal if it is found within easy reach in the EMG laboratory more often than on the library shelf.

Even such a straightforward undertaking as preparation of this handbook is never the work of one person. The staffs of the Department of Neurology of the University of Utah Medical Center, where I did my residency, and the Veterans Administration Medical Center in Salt Lake City were supportive. L. W. Jarcho, M.D., E. T. Ajax, M.D., C. H. Millikan, M.D., J. H. Petajan, M.D., Ph.D., D. J. Thurman, M.D., and F. A. Ziter, M.D., provided much-needed advice and encouragement. Alice Reis typed the many revisions of the handbook, and Linda Broadhead assisted in typing the final manuscript. Dana Crisp skillfully transformed my rough sketches into finished illustrations, and Keith Johnson provided the important photographic support.

L. L. T.

The Electromyographer's Handbook

Chapter 1: Introduction to Nerve Conduction Studies

Nerve conduction studies are commonly used in the evaluation of suspected neuromuscular disease. They are easily performed, and the results obtained in different laboratories are consistent. However, attention to the details of the technique is critical in arriving at accurate latency, amplitude, duration, and configuration determinations. The general approach to the performance of nerve conduction studies is presented in this chapter; specific studies are detailed in the chapters that follow.

Stimulation of a nerve at a single point provides a *latency* measurement. A latency is the time in milliseconds from the stimulus artifact to the recorded response. If a motor nerve can be stimulated at two separate points, two latencies can be obtained and a *nerve conduction velocity* (NCV) calculated.

$$\text{NCV (meters/second)} = \frac{\text{Distance from point 1 to point 2 (millimeters)}}{\text{Latency 2 (milliseconds)} - \text{Latency 1 (milliseconds)}}$$

For example:

Latency 1: 3.0 msec
Latency 2: 6.0 msec
Distance from point 1 to point 2 = 200 mm

$$\text{NCV} = \frac{200 \text{ mm}}{6 \text{ msec} - 3 \text{ msec}} = \frac{200 \text{ mm}}{3 \text{ msec}} = 66.7 \text{ m/second}$$

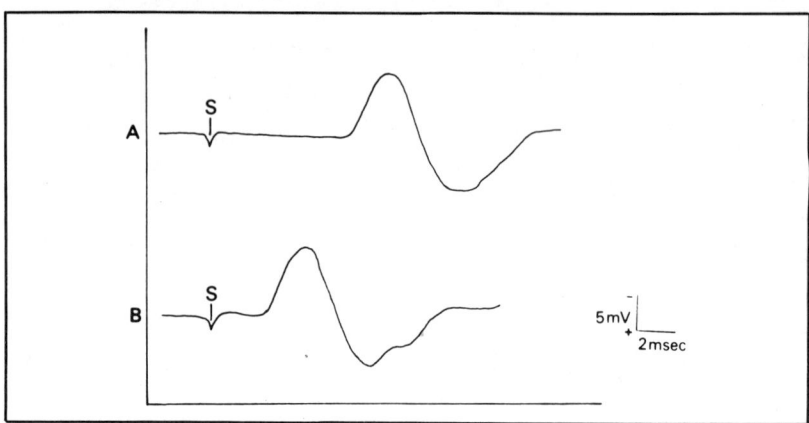

Figure 1-1
Evoked muscle action potentials from the abductor pollicis brevis following stimulation of the median nerve in the antecubital fossa (A) and at the wrist (B).

Since there is no synapse involved in sensory nerve measurements, a conduction velocity can be calculated using a single latency and the distance between the stimulating and recording electrodes. However, the latency and distance are often simply reported alone.

MOTOR STUDIES

Motor nerve measurements involve stimulating an accessible nerve and recording the *evoked muscle action potential* (EMAP) from an appropriate muscle (Fig. 1-1).

In motor nerve conduction studies it is necessary to use a supramaximal stimulus. This procedure ensures that the fascicles containing the fastest conducting fibers are stimulated to avoid incorrectly long latency measurements [2]. To ensure a supramaximal stimulus the voltage should be increased to at least 25 percent greater than that above which no increase in amplitude of the EMAP is seen.

In the determination of motor latencies, the onset of the initial negative (upward) deflection from the baseline is the point that determines latency. Please note that the convention used throughout this handbook is that upward potentials on the oscilloscope are negative and downward potentials are positive. When the recording electrode is negative relative to the reference electrode, the recorded potential is upward. This initial upward deflection can be more exactly determined by using the fastest sweep speed (i.e., fewer milliseconds per centimeter) that allows the onset of the potential to be recorded. The usual oscilloscope will have a 10 × 10-cm screen. Therefore, if the latency being measured is less than 10 msec, a setting of 1 msec per centimeter can be used in making the latency measurement. However, a longer time per division setting is used initially so that the entire EMAP may be visualized and its amplitude and configuration appreciated. Also, the amplification or gain (millivolts per centimeter) should be set so that the entire EMAP can be seen. The amplitude is measured from the baseline to the peak of the negative deflection.

In recording an evoked action potential from a muscle, negativity represents the site of depolarization. If the recording electrode is at a distance from the center of depolarization, the initial deflection becomes positive. Surface electrodes placed over large muscle groups record potential changes that represent an average of the potential changes within that group of muscles. For example, a surface electrode placed over the gastrocnemius will record potential changes within the gastrocnemius and soleus resulting from supramaximal stimulation of the posterior tibial nerve. This implies that latency measurements will vary with the intensity of stimulation because different combinations of muscles are depolarized at different intensities. To obviate this problem, needle electrodes are used to record from muscles other than those of the hands and feet. The needle tip should be repositioned until the initial deflection of the EMAP is negative. Latency measurements to that muscle will then be independent of stimulus intensity, although the amplitude of the evoked response will increase until the maximal level of stimulus intensity is reached.

Sensory nerve studies involve recording the response from the nerve—the *evoked sensory action potential* (ESAP)—at an appropriate distance from the point of stimulation (Fig. 1-2).

SENSORY STUDIES

In the determination of sensory latencies, one measures from the baseline to the *peak* of the negative deflection, rather than to the initial point of negative deflection. The amplitude is also measured to the peak of the negative deflection. With very low amplitude sensory potentials, the 2 msec-per-division setting may allow identification of a potential which is difficult to separate from baseline with a setting of 1 msec per

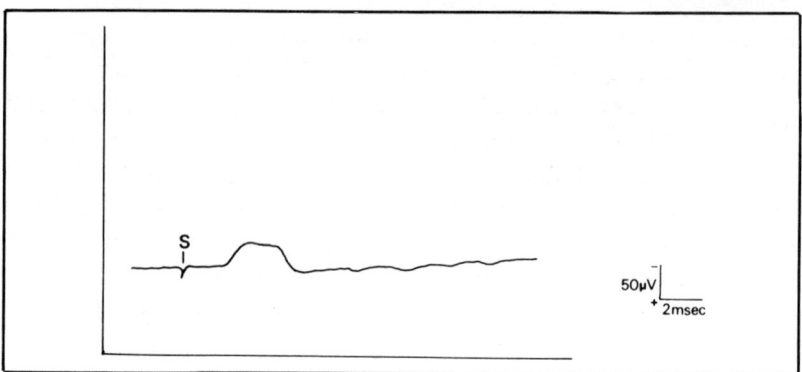

Figure 1-2
Evoked sensory action potential recorded from the median nerve.

division. An on-line signal averager may also be helpful in the positive identification of low amplitude potentials. In sensory nerve lesions proximal to the dorsal root ganglion (i.e., root lesions), sensory latencies remain normal because the distal axon has not been separated from its cell body.

In sensory measurements, sensory nerve action potentials are recorded that are of much lower amplitude than the evoked muscle action potentials recorded in motor studies. A supramaximal stimulus is used, but the threshold stimulus and the supramaximal stimulus are closer in voltage. Care must be taken to avoid contamination of the sensory recording by muscle action potential "artifact," especially when using antidromic stimulation techniques.

In primary myelin degeneration, slowing of conduction velocity is the most prominent electrophysiological disturbance, but increased duration, reduced amplitude, and an increase in the number of phases of the EMAP may also be seen. In primary axonal failure, motor unit potential changes recorded during EMG needle examination of muscle are most prominent, although with severe axonal loss it may be impossible to evoke a muscle action potential or its amplitude may be reduced. Some neuropathies cause varying mixtures of these findings [5].

The following terminology is used in describing the various stimulating and recording electrodes:

Stimulating electrodes
   Cathode: black; solid circle
   Anode: red or white; open circle

Recording electrodes
   Recording electrode: G_1; black; solid circle
   Reference electrode: G_2; red or white; open circle

These electrodes are illustrated in Fig. 1-3. The large disc electrode can be used as a ground. It can also be used as a reference electrode if a monopolar needle electrode is used as the recording electrode (G_1). Types of needle electrodes are discussed in the section on electromyography in Chapter 18.

In general, the G_1 electrode is placed over the motor point [4] of the muscle (see Appendix IX) or over the nerve whose action potential is to be recorded; the G_2 electrode is placed distal to G_1. The cathode is then situated distal to the anode at the point of motor nerve stimulation because stimulation occurs from the cathode (Fig. 1-4). Remember, "black to black." Exceptions to this general rule are noted as they occur.

Nerves are usually stimulated percutaneously but can be stimulated transcutaneously with a needle electrode for such relatively inaccessible nerves as the sciatic and femoral nerves [3]. A percutaneous mode of stimulation is assumed throughout this handbook unless otherwise specified.

Two stimulation points are used in common for many nerves. The first is Erb's point, which is located just above the clavicle in the angle between the posterior border of the clavicular head of the sternocleidomastoid muscle and the clavicle itself at the level of the sixth cervical vertebra. Distances from Erb's point should be measured with obstetrical calipers (Fig. 1-5).

The other common stimulation point is in the axilla and is located in the groove between the coracobrachialis and the medial edge of the brachial triceps, about 18 cm (in the adult) proximal to the medial epicondyle of the humerus. The axillary-brachial artery should be palpable at this point (Fig. 1-6).

Orthodromic stimulation refers to the usual direction of impulse conduction along a nerve: the direction is from distal to proximal along a sensory nerve or from proximal to distal along a motor nerve. *Antidromic* refers to the direction opposite physiological conduction along a nerve. Motor nerve conduction studies are performed orthodromically (stimulate proximally, record distally) whereas sensory studies can be performed either orthodromically (stimulate distally, record proximally) or antidromically (stimulate proximally, record distally).

6

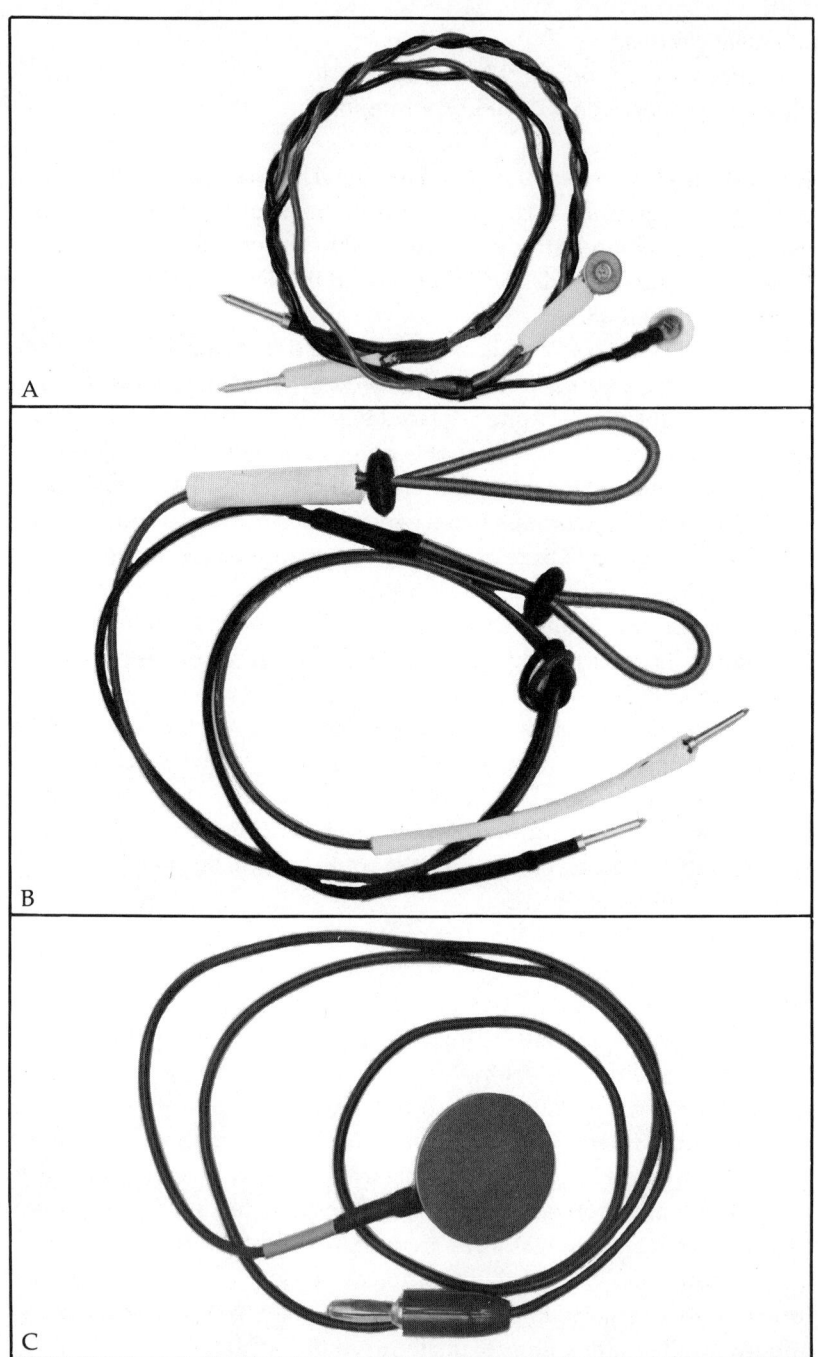

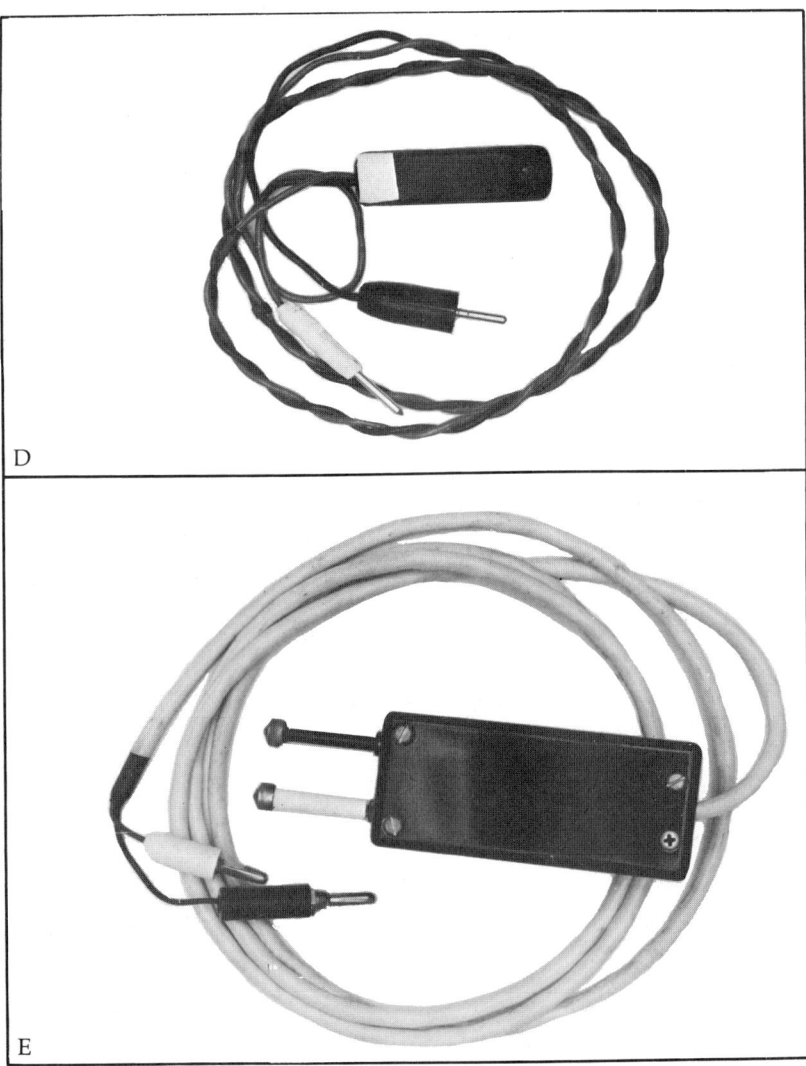

Figure 1-3
Types of surface electrodes. Note that the anodal and/or G_2 electrodes have been marked with white tape. (This marking is used for clarity in the photographs of electrode placement.) A. Small disc recording electrodes. B. Ring electrodes. C. Large disc electrode. D. Bipolar electrode. E. Hand-held bipolar stimulation electrode.

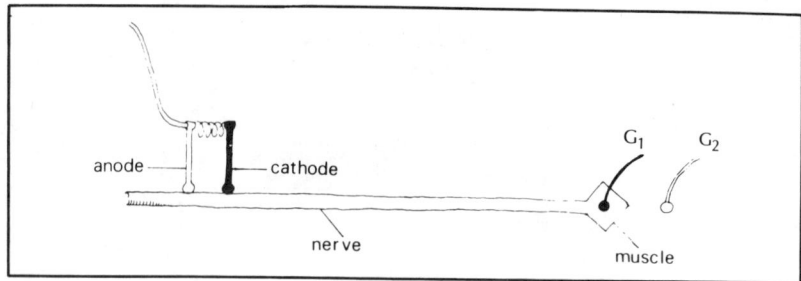

Figure 1-4
Diagrammatic electrode placement for motor nerve stimulation.

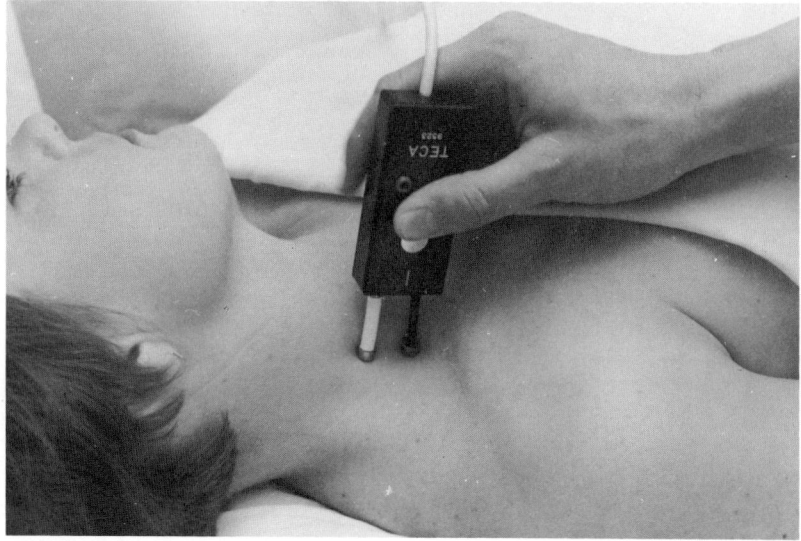

Figure 1-5
Stimulation at Erb's point.

9   1. Introduction to Nerve Conduction Studies

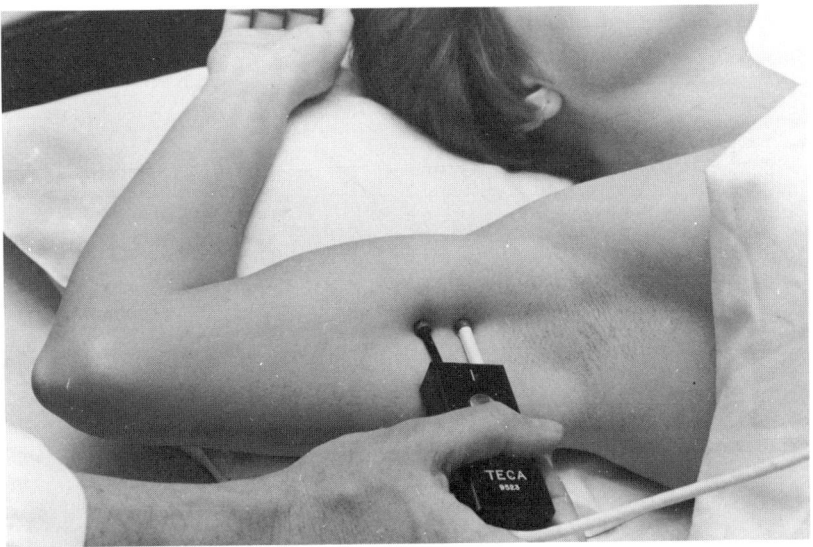

Figure 1-6
Stimulation in the axilla.

In recording results of nerve stimulation, it is best to record not only latency, but also amplitude and configuration (with a drawing or photograph) of the ESAP or EMAP. Results from various sources are not always in exact agreement. Therefore, it is important for each laboratory to determine a normal value for each procedure. The average motor conduction velocity in the upper extremity is 60 m per second and the average motor conduction velocity in the lower extremity is 45 m per second. Values in the newborn [1] are about one-half those of the adult, reaching adult values at the age of four years (Table 1-1). The normal range for sensory latencies is approximately 2 to 3.5 msec.

The formal EMG report should include: (1) the name of the nerve studied; (2) the direction of stimulation (orthodromic or antidromic); (3) the points of stimulation; (4) the distal latency, the proximal latency or latencies as appropriate; (5) the amplitudes of the evoked potentials; (6) the distance(s) between points of stimulation; and (7) conduction velocity when calculated.

In the chapters that follow, a discussion of relevant anatomy and commonly suggested applications precedes the details of the procedure

Table 1-1
Motor Nerve Conduction Velocities at Different Ages

Average Age of Group (weeks)	Ulnar (m/sec)	Median (m/sec)	Peroneal (m/sec)	Posterior Tibial (m/sec)
5	34.5	33.1	37.2	34.3
18	35.4	35.8	39.1	32.7
34	46.1	41.8	44.1	38.3
56	46.7	40.4	46.7	39.8
88	51.6	47.5	49.5	44.5
140	52.4	49.4	44.2	43.1
210	56.1	54.9	52.2	48.4

Source: Adapted from R. D. Baer and E. W. Johnson. Motor nerve conduction velocities in normal children. *Arch. Phys. Med. Rehabil.* October: 698, 1965. Used by permission.

and the compilations of expected values. For some nerves both motor and sensory studies are easily done and both are described. For other nerves only a motor technique or a sensory technique has been well standardized and only that study is discussed.

REFERENCES

1. Baer, D., and Johnson, E. W. Motor nerve conduction velocities in normal children. *Arch. Phys. Med. Rehabil.* October:698, 1965.
2. Goodgold, J., and Eberstein, A. *Electrodiagnosis of Neuromuscular Diseases* (2nd ed.). Baltimore: Williams & Wilkins, 1977.
3. Lambert, E. H., and Daube, R. (Chairmen). *Special Course #16: Clinical Electromyography.* American Academy of Neurology Meeting, Chicago, Ill., April 23–28, 1979.
4. Licht, S. (Ed.). *Electrodiagnosis and Electromyography* (3rd ed.). New Haven: Licht, 1971.
5. Liveson, J. A., and Spielholz, N. I. *Peripheral Neurology.* Philadelphia: Davis, 1979.

ADDITIONAL READING

Cohen, H. L., and Brumlick, J. *A Manual of Electroneuromyography* (2nd ed.). Hagerstown, Md.: Harper & Row, 1976.

Goodgold, J. *Anatomical Correlates of Clinical Electromyography.* Baltimore: Williams & Wilkins, 1974.

Goodgold, J., and Eberstein, A. *Electrodiagnosis of Neuromuscular Diseases* (2nd ed.). Baltimore: Williams & Wilkins, 1977.

Johnson, E. W. (Ed.). *Practical Electromyography.* Baltimore: Williams & Wilkins, 1980.

Kopell, H. P., and Thompson, W. A. L. *Peripheral Entrapment Neuropathies.* Baltimore: Williams & Wilkins, 1963.

Lenman, J. A. R., and Ritchie, A. E. *Clinical Electromyography* (2nd ed.). Bath: Pitman, 1977.

Licht, S. (Ed.). *Electrodiagnosis and Electromyography* (3rd ed.). New Haven: Licht, 1971.

Liveson, J. A., and Spielholz, N. I. *Peripheral Neurology.* Philadelphia: Davis, 1979.

Remond, A. (Ed.). *Handbook of Electroencephalography and Clinical Neurophysiology—Volume 16* (F. Buchthal [Ed.]): *Electromyography.* Amsterdam: Elsevier, 1975.

Riddoch, Brigadier G. (Chairman). *Aids to the Investigation of Peripheral Nerve Injuries* (2nd ed.). London: Her Majesty's Stationery Office, 1943.

Smorto, M. P., and Basmajian, J. V. *Electrodiagnosis.* Hagerstown, Md.: Harper & Row, 1977.

Smorto, M. P., and Basmajian, J. V. *Clinical Electroneurography* (2nd ed.). Baltimore: Williams & Wilkins, 1979.

Walton, J. N. (Ed.). *Disorders of Voluntary Muscle* (3rd ed.). Edinburgh: Churchill Livingstone, 1974.

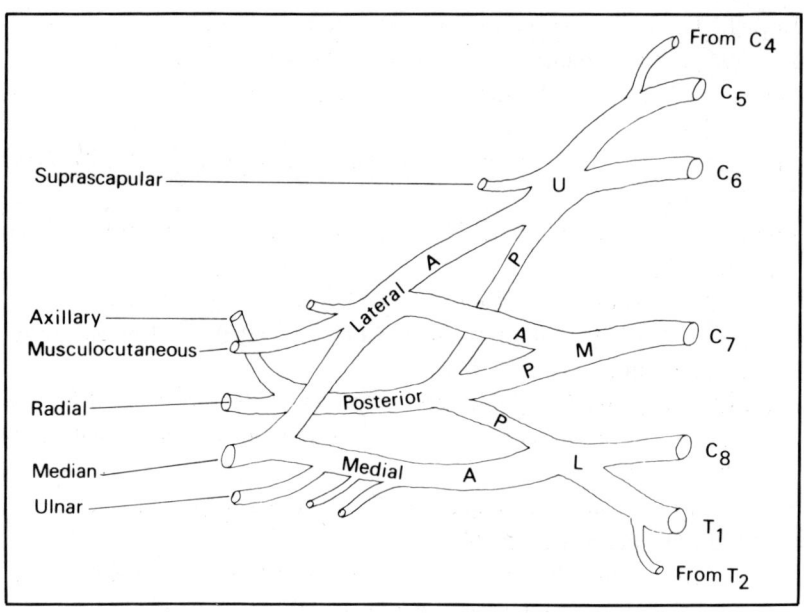

Figure 2-1
Simplified plan of the brachial plexus emphasizing commonly studied nerves. (U, M, L = upper, middle, and lower trunks. A, P = anterior and posterior divisions of each trunk; lateral, medial, posterior cords.)

Chapter 2 Brachial Plexus
(Motor Studies)

ANATOMY

The *brachial plexus* is composed of the anterior (ventral) primary rami (divisions) of *spinal nerves* originating from spinal segments $C_{5,6,7,8}$ and T_1 (Fig. 2-1). In the lower part of the neck these ventral rami pass between the scalenus anterior and scalenus medius muscles. The five ventral rami merge into three trunks that run obliquely downwards and laterally to pass as a compact bundle over the first rib and behind the middle third of the clavicle to enter the axilla. Each trunk divides into anterior and posterior divisions that then unite to form three cords from which most of the peripheral nerves to the upper limb are ultimately formed. It should be noted that the ventral ramus (division) of a spinal nerve contains fibers from both the ventral (anterior) motor and dorsal (posterior) sensory roots of the spinal nerve that attach it to the spinal cord.

APPLICATIONS

The proximal shoulder girdle muscles may be involved initially in such diverse conditions as brachial plexus neuritis, polyneuritis, cervical disc herniation, anterior horn cell disease, myasthenic syndromes, and nerve entrapment syndromes such as the one involving the suprascapular nerve. Early in their presentation some of these conditions may be difficult to differentiate clinically. Latency measurements can clarify some of these problems [1]. Early in their courses, anterior horn cell disease, root lesions, and myasthenia gravis do not affect the latency values, but an increase in latency suggests a demyelinating nerve trunk lesion at or distal to Erb's point.

The best site for stimulation of the trunks of the brachial plexus is at Erb's point, which is located just above the clavicle in the angle between the posterior edge of the sternocleidomastoid muscle and the clavicle itself at the level of the sixth cervical vertebra (Fig. 1-5). (The place of origin of the suprascapular nerve from the upper trunk of the brachial plexus is also known as Erb's point.)

The proximal muscles from which it is easiest to record evoked muscle potentials are biceps (musculocutaneous nerve), supraspinatus and infraspinatus (suprascapular nerve), deltoid (circumflex nerve), and triceps (radial nerve). The recording needle electrodes (G_1) must be placed in the belly of each muscle, sometimes at different levels along a vertical line in the middle of a single muscle in order to obtain several responses. Distances from Erb's point to G_1 are measured with calipers.

PROCEDURE

1. Electrode placement
    a. G_1 recording electrode over the muscle to be tested
    b. G_2 recording electrode distal to G_1 over a bony prominence, when possible
    c. Ground plate between the stimulating and recording electrodes
2. Stimulation: Erb's point (Fig. 1-5)

NORMAL MEAN LATENCIES

(Values taken from Gassel [1].)

Muscle	Distance from Erb's point (cm)	Latency (SD in msec)
Biceps brachii	20.0	4.6 ± 0.6
(Fig. 2-2)	24.0	4.7 ± 0.6
	28.0	5.0 ± 0.5
Deltoid	15.5	4.3 ± 0.5
(Fig. 2-3)	18.5	4.4 ± 0.35
Triceps brachii	21.5	4.5 ± 0.42
(Fig. 2-4)	26.5	4.9 ± 0.45
	31.5	5.3 ± 0.32
Supraspinatus	8.5	2.6 ± 0.32
(Fig. 2-5)	10.5	2.7 ± 0.27
Infraspinatus	14.0	3.4 ± 0.4
(Fig. 2-6)	17.0	3.4 ± 0.5

2. Brachial Plexus

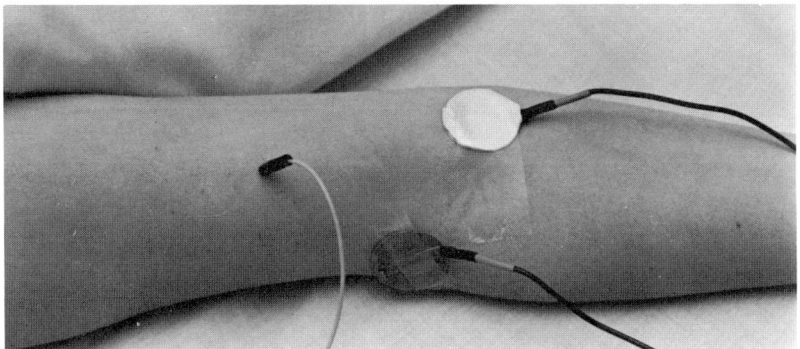

Figure 2-2
Placement of recording electrodes for study of the biceps brachii.

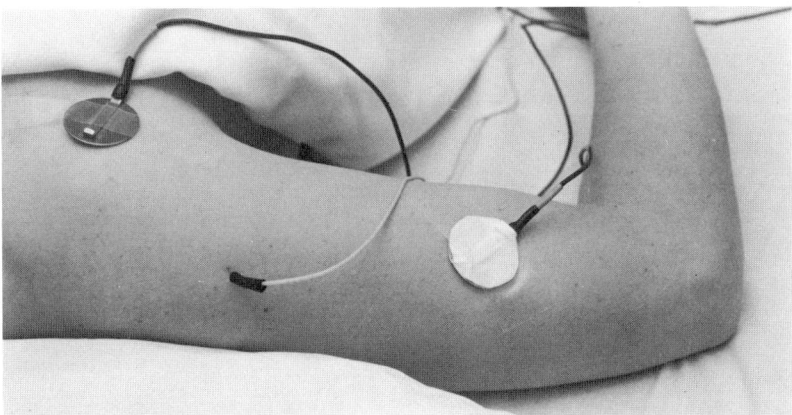

Figure 2-3
Placement of recording electrodes for study of the deltoid.

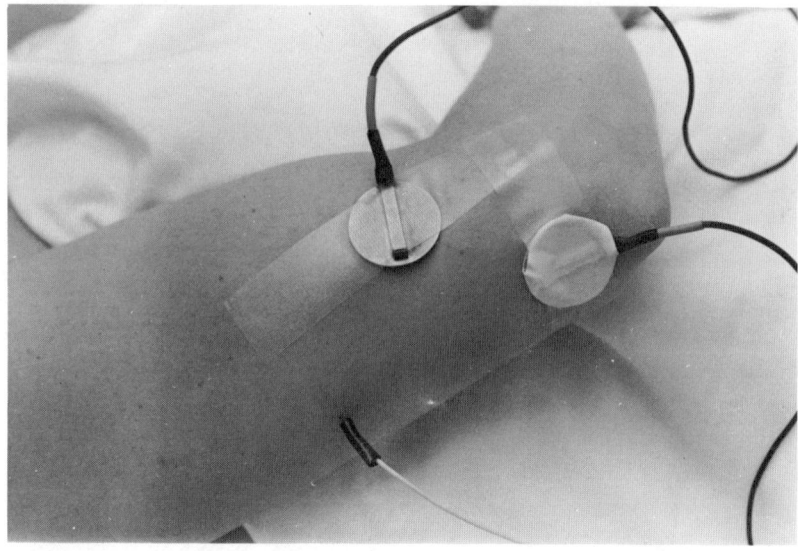

Figure 2-4
Placement of recording electrodes for study of the triceps.

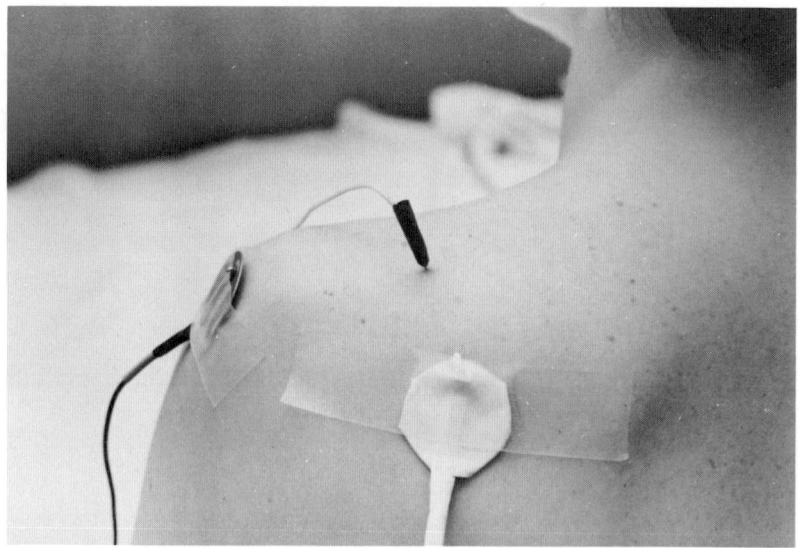

Figure 2-5
Placement of recording electrodes for study of the supraspinatus.

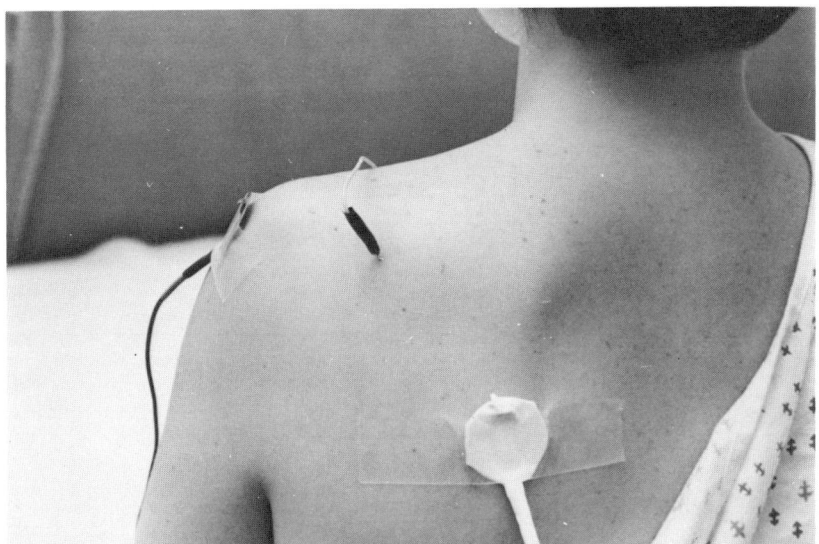

Figure 2-6
Placement of recording electrodes for study of the infraspinatus.

REFERENCE

1. Gassel, M. M. A test of nerve conduction to the muscles of the shoulder girdle in the diagnosis of proximal neurogenic and muscular disease. *J. Neurol. Neurosurg. Psychiatry* 27:200, 1964.

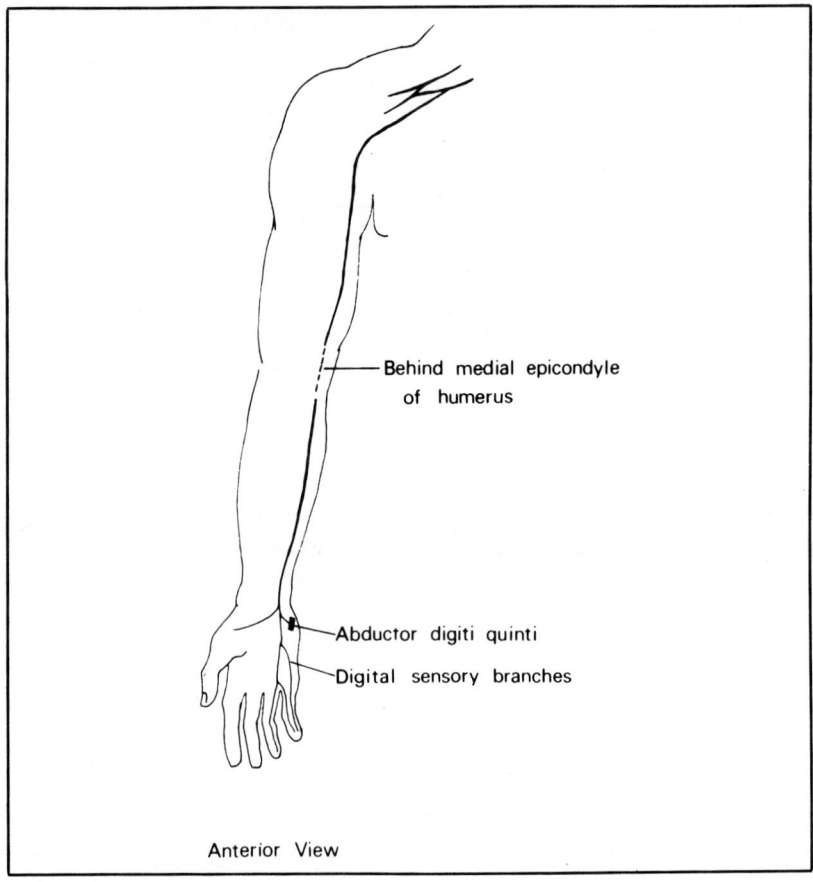

Figure 3-1
Origin and course of the ulnar nerve.

Chapter 3

Ulnar Nerve
(Motor and Sensory Studies)

ANATOMY

The *ulnar nerve* is the motor nerve to the muscles of the ulnar side of the forearm and hand and the sensory nerve to the skin of the ulnar aspect of hand, the fifth digit, and the ulnar half of the fourth digit (Fig. 3-1). It receives contributions from C_8 and T_1, which pass through the lower trunk and medial cord of the *brachial plexus* to occupy a superficial position along the medial side of the arm and forearm as the ulnar nerve.

APPLICATIONS

The ulnar nerve may be involved in compressive lesions in the hand, wrist, elbow, and thoracic outlet. The lower trunk and medial cord of the brachial plexus are in close proximity to the first rib.

PROCEDURE (MOTOR)

1. Electrode placement (Fig. 3-2)
   a. G_1 over the midportion of the abductor digiti quinti
   b. G_2 over proximal phalanx of fifth digit
   c. Ground over dorsum of hand between G_1 and G_2 (Fig. 3-3)
2. Stimulation
   a. Palmar aspect of wrist over medial distal ulna with the cathode 5.5 cm proximal to G_1 (Fig. 3-2)
   b. Just distal to the osseous groove in the posterior aspect of the medial epicondyle of the humerus, that is, the ulnar groove (Fig. 3-4)
   c. Just proximal to the ulnar groove (Fig. 3-5)

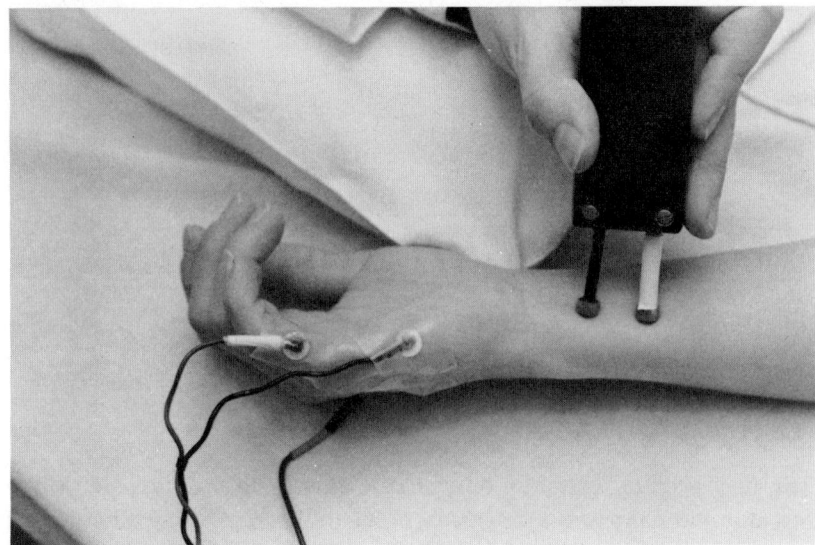

Figure 3-2
Electrode placement for recording from the abductor digiti quinti and stimulation of the ulnar nerve at the wrist.

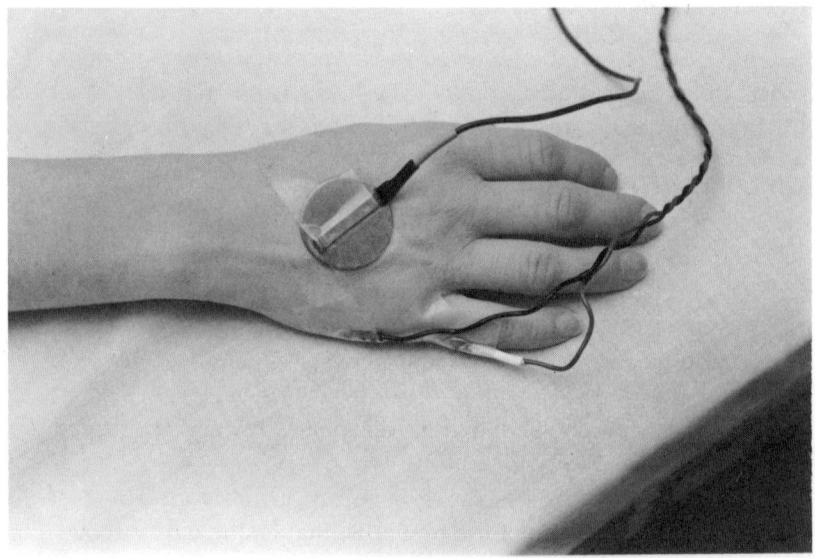

Figure 3-3
Placement of the ground on the dorsum of the hand.

3. Ulnar Nerve

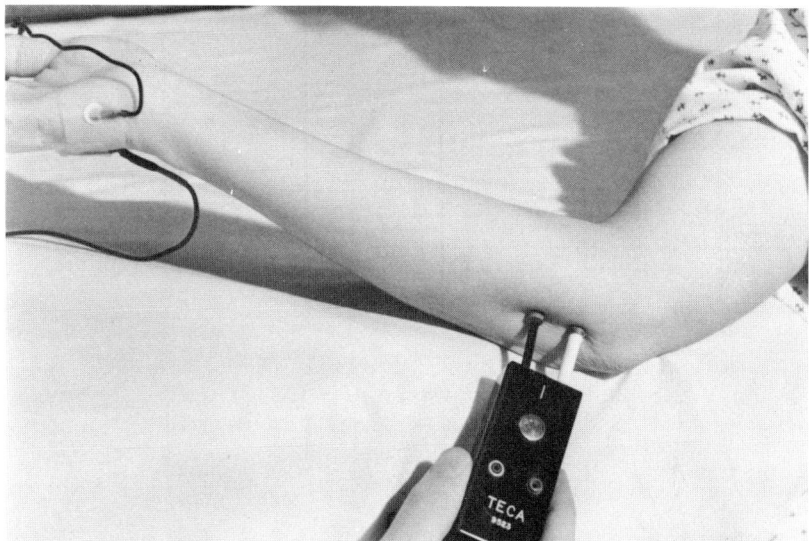

Figure 3-4
Stimulation of the ulnar nerve just distal to the ulnar groove.

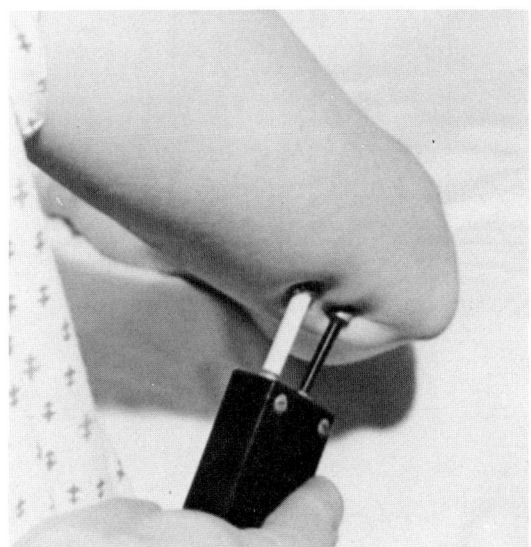

Figure 3-5
Stimulation of the ulnar nerve just proximal to the ulnar groove.

d. Axilla (see Fig. 1-6)
e. Erb's point (see Fig. 1-5)

NORMAL VALUES (MOTOR)

Segment	Distal Latency or NCV	Amplitude (mV)	Reference
Wrist to abductor digiti quinti	3.5 ± 0.36 (2.8–4.2) msec	11.3 (6–16)	[2, 3]
Below elbow to wrist	48.9 ± 2.8 (45.2–55.3) m/sec	11.3 (6–16)	[2, 3]
Above elbow to wrist	48.9 ± 2.8 (45.2–55.3) m/sec	11.3 (6–16)	[2, 3]
Axilla to above elbow	51.2 ± 4.2 (44.9–60.6) m/sec	11.3 (6–16)	[2, 3]
Erb's to axilla	63.0 ± 5.5 (55.0–73.2) m/sec	11.3 (6–16)	[2, 3]
Erb's to above elbow	60.1 ± 4.8 (51.0–72.9) m/sec	11.3 (6–16)	[3, 4, 5]

PROCEDURE (SENSORY; ORTHODROMIC)

1. Place the ring cathode around the fifth digit near the metacarpophalangeal joint (Fig. 3-6).
2. Place the ring anode around the fifth distal interphalangeal joint.
3. Locate the ground on the dorsum of the hand "between" G_1 and G_2.
4. Locate the G_1 end of the recording dual electrode over the ulnar nerve at the wrist 13 cm from the ring cathode.

NORMAL VALUES (SENSORY; ORTHODROMIC)

Age (years)	Amplitude (μV)	Sensory Latency (msec)	Reference
...	...	2.8 ± 0.2	[6]
18–25	> 2 (mean 13)	...	[1]
70–79	> 2 (mean 5)	...	[1]

3. Ulnar Nerve

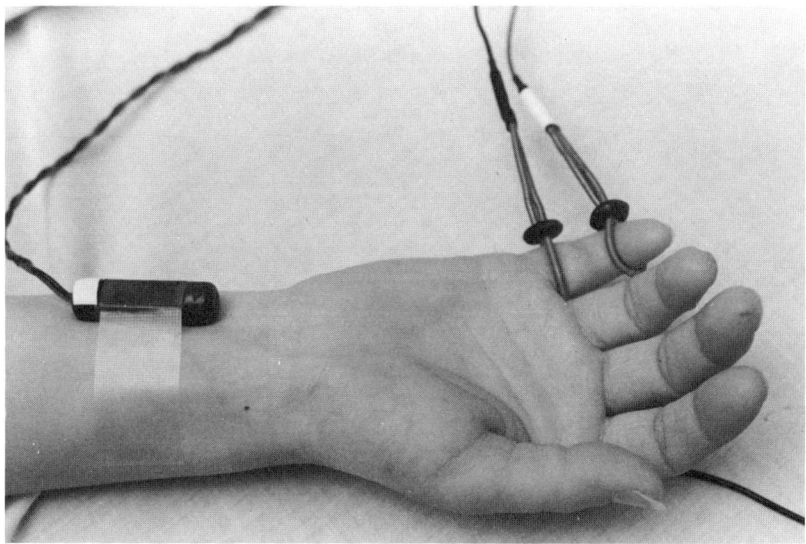

Figure 3-6
Electrode placement for orthodromic sensory stimulation of the ulnar nerve.

PROCEDURE (SENSORY; ANTIDROMIC)

1. Place the G_1 ring electrode around the fifth digit near the metacarpophalangeal joint (Fig. 3-7).
2. Place the G_2 ring electrode around the fifth digit near the distal interphalangeal joint.
3. Locate the ground on the dorsum of the hand.
4. Stimulate the ulnar nerve at the wrist with the cathode 13 cm proximal to the G_1 ring electrode.

NORMAL VALUES (SENSORY; ANTIDROMIC)

Amplitude	Sensory Latency (msec)	Reference
Same or slightly higher than orthodromic	3.2 ± 0.3	[7]

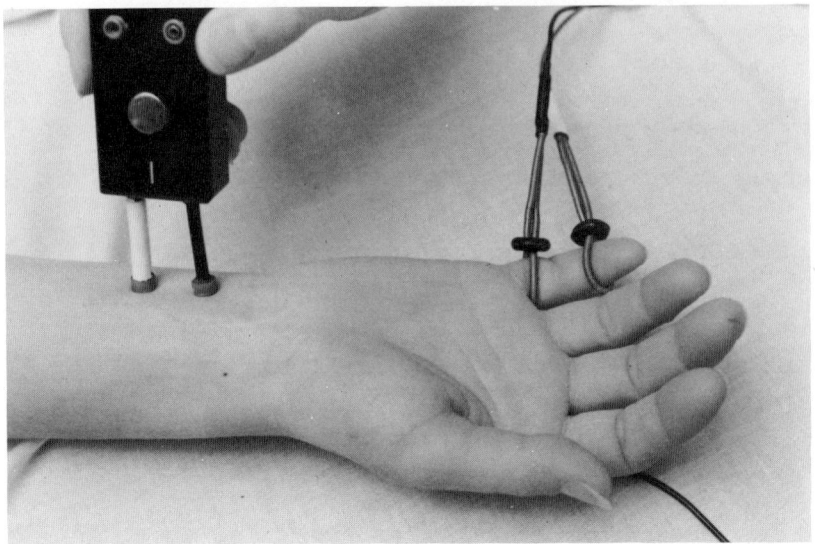

Figure 3-7
Electrode placement for antidromic sensory stimulation of the ulnar nerve.

REFERENCES

1. Buchthal, F., and Rosenfalck, A. Evoked action potentials and conduction velocity in human sensory nerves. *Brain Res.* 3:1, 1966.
2. Ginzburg, M., Lee, M., Ginzburg, J., and Alba, A. Median and ulnar nerve conduction determinations in the Erb's point-axilla segment in normal subjects. *J. Neurol. Neurosurg. Psychiatry* 41:444, 1978.
3. Hodes, R., Larrabee, M. G., and German, W. The human electromyogram in response to nerve stimulation and conduction velocity of motor axons. *Arch. Neurol. Psychiatry* 60:340, 1948.
4. Jebsen, R. H. Motor conduction velocities in the median and ulnar nerves. *Arch. Phys. Med. Rehabil.* 48:185, 1967.
5. London, G. W. Normal ulnar nerve conduction velocity across the thoracic outlet: Comparison of two measuring techniques. *J. Neurol. Neurosurg. Psychiatry* 38:756, 1975.
6. Mavor, H., and Libman, I. Motor nerve conduction velocity measurement as a diagnostic tool. *Neurology* (Minneap.) 12:733, 1962.
7. Melvin, J. L., Harris, D. H., and Johnson, E. W. Sensory and motor conduction velocities in the ulnar and median nerves. *Arch. Phys. Med. Rehabil.* 47:511, 1966.

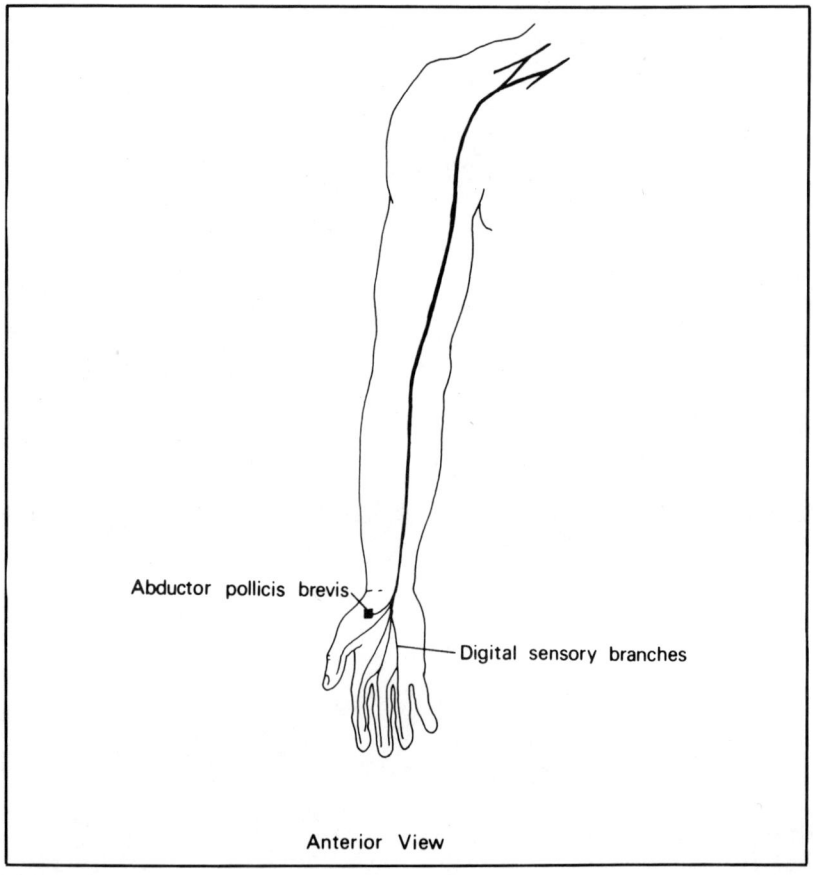

Figure 4-1
Origin and course of the median nerve.

Chapter 4 Median Nerve
(Motor and Sensory Studies)

ANATOMY

The *median nerve* serves mainly as the motor nerve to the radial side of the flexor portion of the forearm and the muscles of the thenar eminence and as the sensory nerve to the radial (lateral) palmar surface including all or part of the palmar surfaces of the first four digits (Fig. 4-1). The median nerve receives fibers from $C_{6,7,8,}$ and T_1, which pass through the upper, middle, and lower trunks of the *brachial plexus* into the lateral and medial cords, the terminal portions of which merge to form the median nerve. The median nerve then descends in the upper arm in close proximity to the brachial artery and finally traverses the midventral aspect of the forearm to the tunnel under the flexor retinaculum (carpal tunnel) from which it emerges to innervate the LOAF muscles of the hand (first and second *l*umbricals, *o*pponens pollicis, *a*bductor pollicis brevis, and *f*lexor pollicis brevis).

APPLICATIONS

The median nerve is commonly entrapped in the carpal tunnel. It is less frequently involved in the pronator syndrome, anterior interosseous syndrome, and the ligament of Struther's syndrome [5]. Rarely, compression of the brachial plexus in the thoracic outlet may involve nerve fibers that ultimately join the median nerve.

PROCEDURE (MOTOR)

1. Electrode placement (Fig. 4.2)
   a. G_1 over the abductor pollicis brevis

b. G_2 over proximal phalanx of the thumb
   c. Ground over dorsum of hand, between G_1 and G_2
2. Stimulation
   a. Palmar aspect, midwrist, with the cathode 5.5 cm proximal to G_1 (Fig. 4-2)
   b. Elbow (antecubital fossa) just medial to the palpable brachial artery (Fig. 4-3)
   c. Axilla (Fig. 1-6)
   d. Erb's point (Fig. 1-5)

NORMAL VALUES (MOTOR)

Segment	Distal Latency or NCV	Amplitude (mV)	Reference
Wrist to abductor pollicis brevis	3.9 ± 0.37 (3.4–4.5) msec	11.8 (7–17)	[2, 3]
Elbow to wrist	49.0 ± 3.9 (45.1–54.4) m/sec	11.8 (7–17)	[2, 3]
Axilla to elbow	56.3 ± 5.1 (50.0–68.3) m/sec	11.8 (7–17)	[2, 3]
Erb's to axilla	65.1 ± 6.1 (57.1–76.2) m/sec	11.8 (7–17)	[2, 3]
Erb's to elbow	62.9 ± 6.0 (51.0–76.0) m/sec	11.8 (7–17)	[3, 4]

PROCEDURE (SENSORY; ORTHODROMIC)

1. Place the ring cathode around the second digit near the metacarpophalangeal joint (Fig. 4-4).
2. Place the ring anode around the second digit near the distal interphalangeal joint.
3. Locate the G_1 end of the recording dual electrode over the median nerve on the anterior aspect of the wrist 13 cm proximal to the ring cathode.
4. Place ground on dorsum of hand.

4. Median Nerve

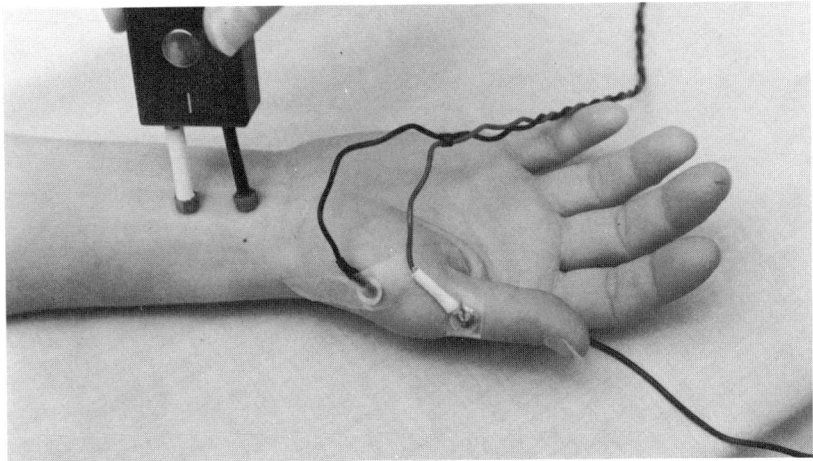

Figure 4-2
Electrode placement for recording from the abductor pollicis brevis and stimulation of the median nerve at the wrist.

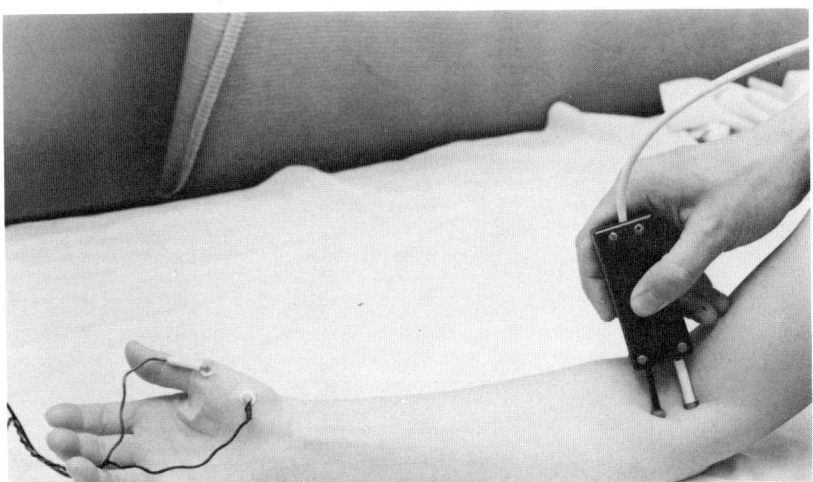

Figure 4-3
Stimulation of the median nerve in the antecubital fossa.

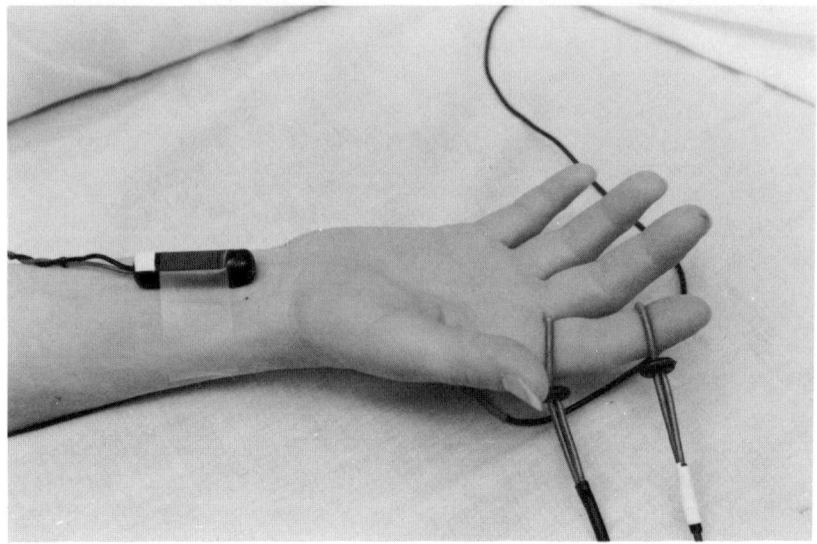

Figure 4-4
Electrode placement for orthodromic sensory stimulation of the median nerve.

NORMAL VALUES (SENSORY; ORTHODROMIC)

Age (years)	Amplitude (μV)	Sensory Latency (msec)	Reference
...	...	3.0 ± 0.25	[6]
18–25	> 11 (mean 25)	...	[1]
40–61	> 7 (mean 12)	...	[1]
70–78	> 4 (mean 8)	...	[1]

PROCEDURE (SENSORY; ANTIDROMIC)

1. Place the G_1 ring around the second digit near the metacarpophalangeal joint (Fig. 4-5).
2. Place the G_2 ring around the second digit near the distal interphalangeal joint.
3. Place ground on dorsum of hand.
4. Stimulate the median nerve (dorsum, midwrist) with the cathode 13 cm proximal to the G_1 ring electrode.

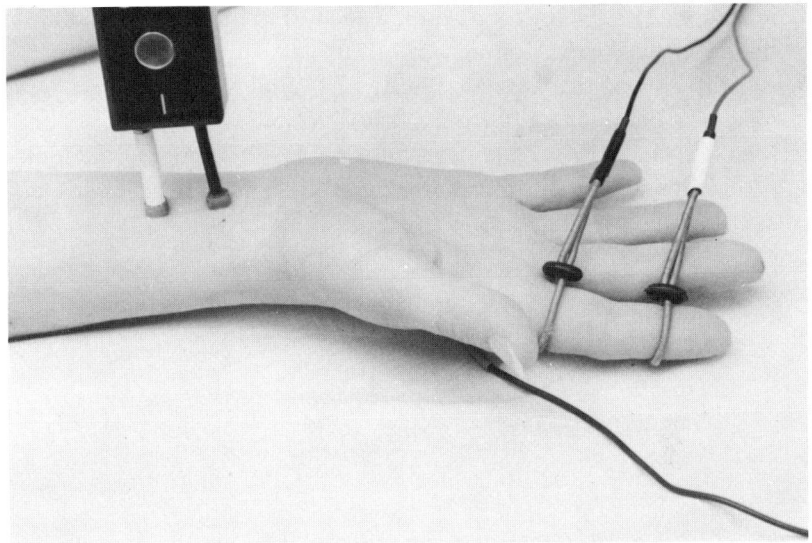

Figure 4-5
Electrode placement for antidromic sensory stimulation of the median nerve.

NORMAL VALUES (SENSORY; ANTIDROMIC)

Amplitude	Sensory Latency (msec)	Reference
Equal to or slightly higher than orthodromic	3.2 ± 0.25	[6]

REFERENCES

1. Buchthal, F., and Rosenfalck, A. Evoked action potentials and conduction velocity in human sensory nerves. *Brain Res.* 3:1, 1966.
2. Ginzburg, M., Lee, M., Ginzburg, J., and Alba, A. Median and ulnar nerve conduction determinations in the Erb's point-axilla segment in normal subjects. *J. Neurol. Neurosurg. Psychiatry* 41:444, 1978.
3. Hodes, R., Larrabee, M. G., and German, W. The human electromyogram in response to nerve stimulation and conduction velocity of motor axons. *Arch. Neurol. Psychiatry* 60:340, 1948.

4. Jebsen, R. H.   Motor conduction velocities in the median and ulnar nerves. *Arch. Phys. Med. Rehabil.* 48:185, 1967.
5. Kopell, P., and Thompson, W. A. L.   *Peripheral Entrapment Neuropathies.* Baltimore: Williams & Wilkins, 1963.
6. Melvin, J. L., Harris, D. H., and Johnson, E. W.   Sensory and motor conduction velocities in the ulnar and median nerves. *Arch. Phys. Med. Rehabil.* 47:511, 1966.

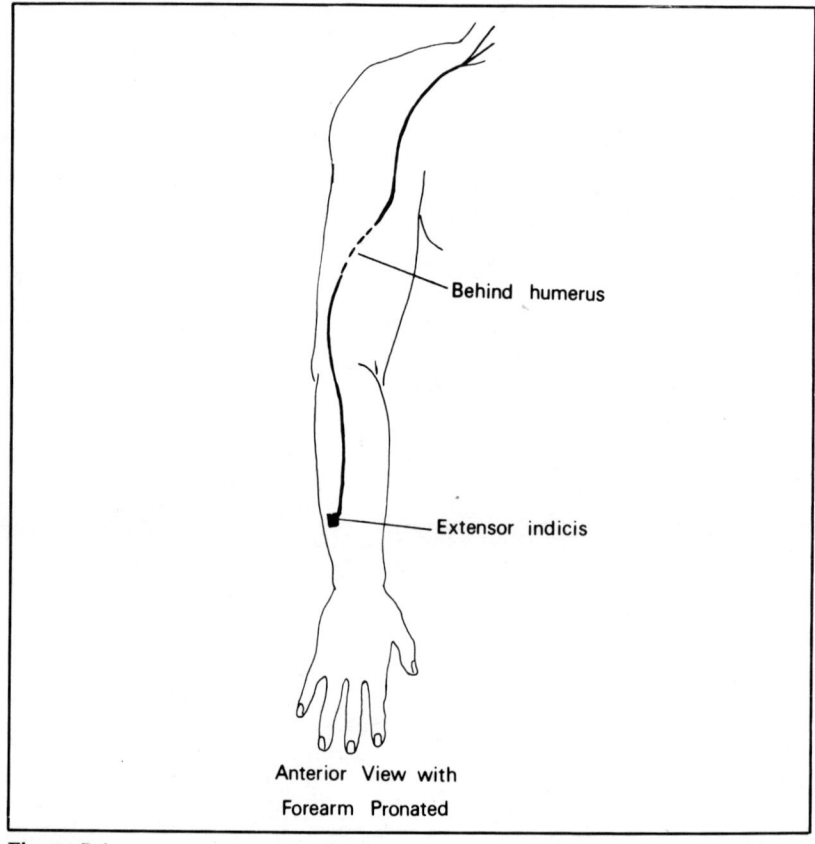

Figure 5-1
Origin and course of the radial nerve. (The superficial sensory radial nerve is shown in Figure 5-4.)

Chapter 5 Radial Nerve
(Motor and Sensory Studies)

ANATOMY

The *radial nerve* receives contributions from $C_{5,6,7,8}$, and variably from T_1. The largest terminal branch of the *brachial plexus*, the radial nerve is the continuation of the posterior cord and supplies the extensor muscles of the arm and forearm (Fig. 5-1) as well as the skin covering them. The radial sensory fibers proper originate from the C_6 or C_7 roots, or both, and pass through the upper or middle trunk, or both, and through the posterior cord. They separate from the deep motor branch near the elbow, and pass distally down the forearm beneath the brachioradialis muscle. In the distal forearm the radial sensory nerve becomes superficial, crosses the radius, and supplies the lateral (radial) aspect of the dorsum of the hand and the proximal dorsum of the first three and one-half digits (see Fig. 5-4).

APPLICATIONS

The radial nerve is involved in "Saturday night" palsies, "tennis elbow," the posterior interosseous syndrome, and "handcuff" neuropathy. Radial conduction studies allow evaluation of the upper and middle trunks and posterior cord of the brachial plexus.

PROCEDURE (MOTOR)

1. Electrode placement (Fig. 5-2)
    a. G_1 over the extensor indicis proprius muscle. The extensor indicis proprius is innervated by the most distal motor branch of the radial nerve. This muscle originates from the dorsal surface of the

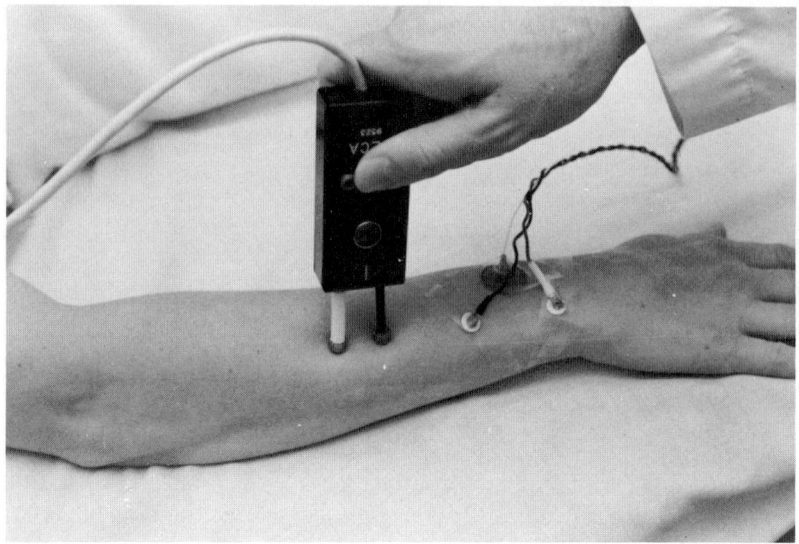

Figure 5-2
Electrode placement for recording from the extensor indicis proprius and distal stimulation of the radial nerve (motor).

body of the ulna below the origin of the extensor pollicis longus and from the interosseous membrane. The distal body of the extensor proprius can be palpated along the dorsal ulnar aspect of the forearm approximately 4 to 6 cm proximal to the ulnar styloid, just lateral (radial) to the ulna. It may be best to confirm this muscle's location with the EMG needle; it is sometimes necessary to record (G_1) from a subcutaneous or intramuscular needle rather than from the usual surface electrode.
  b. Locate G_2 over the ulnar styloid.
  c. Locate ground between G_1 and G_2.
2. Stimulation
  a. In the forearm approximately 8 cm proximal to the ulnar styloid where the radial nerve can be palpated just lateral (radial) to the extensor carpi ulnaris muscle (Fig. 5-2).
  b. At the elbow in the groove between the brachioradialis muscle and the biceps tendon, about 6 cm proximal to the lateral epicondyle of the humerus (Fig. 5-3).
  c. Axilla (see Fig. 1-6).
  d. Erb's point (see Fig. 1-5).

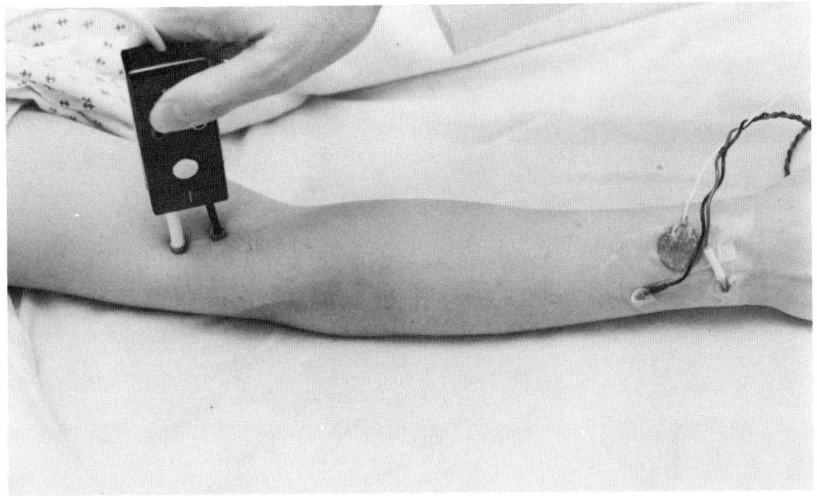

Figure 5-3
Proximal stimulation of the radial nerve (motor) in the antecubital fossa.

NORMAL VALUES (MOTOR)

Segment	Distal Latency or NCV	Amplitude (mV)	Reference
Erb's to elbow	72 (56–93) m/sec	10.5 (8–14)	[1, 2]
Axilla to elbow	69 ± 5.6 m/sec	11 ± 7.0	[1, 4]
Elbow to forearm	62 ± 5.1 m/sec	13 ± 8.2	[4]
Forearm to extensor indicis proprius	2.4 ± 0.5 msec	14 ± 8.8	[4]

The conduction time should be 10 percent faster in the proximal fibers than in the distal fibers.

PROCEDURE (SENSORY; ANTIDROMIC)

1. Locate the superficial (sensory) radial nerve as it crosses the tendon of the extensor pollicis longus on the ulnar side of the anatomic snuffbox. It should be palpable at this crossing point (Fig. 5-4).
2. Place the G_1 electrode over the palpable superficial radial nerve (Fig. 5-5).

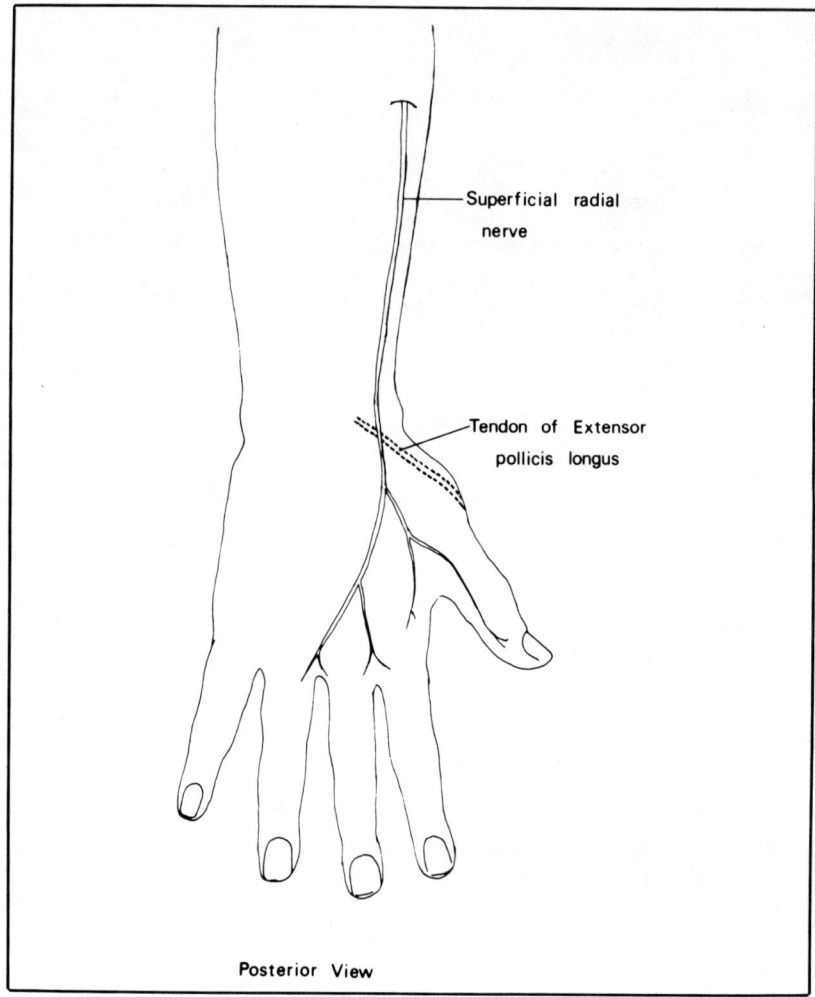

Figure 5-4
Superficial course of the radial sensory nerve.

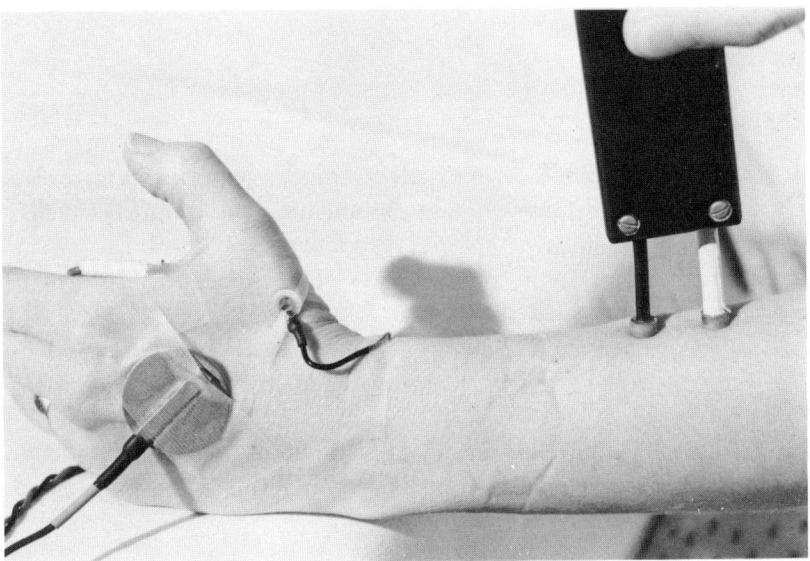

Figure 5-5
Electrode placement for antidromic sensory stimulation of the superficial radial nerve.

3. Place the G_2 electrode 3 cm distal to G_1 over the first dorsal interosseous muscle.
4. Place the ground over the dorsum of the hand "between" the G_1 and G_2 electrodes.
5. Stimulate with the cathode 10 cm proximal to G_1 over the lateral (radial) aspect of the radius.

NORMAL VALUES (SENSORY; ANTIDROMIC)

Age (years)	Amplitude (μV)	Sensory Latency (msec)	Reference
15	> 18 (mean 30)	< 2.6 (mean 2.2)	[3]
65	> 10 (mean 25)	< 2.8 (mean 2.5)	[3]

REFERENCES

1. Hodes, R., Larrabee, M. G., and German, W. The human electromyogram in response to nerve stimulation and conduction velocity of motor axons. *Arch. Neurol. Psychiatry* 60:340, 1948.
2. Jebsen, R. H. Motor conduction velocity in proximal and distal segments of the radial nerve. *Arch. Phys. Med. Rehabil.* 47:597, 1966.
3. Lambert, E. H., and Daube, J. R. (Chairmen). *Special Course #16: Clinical Electromyography.* American Academy of Neurology Meeting, April 23–28, 1979.
4. Trojaborg, W., and Sindrup, G. H. Motor and sensory conduction in different segments of the radial nerve in normal subjects. *J. Neurol. Neurosurg. Psychiatry* 32:354, 1969.

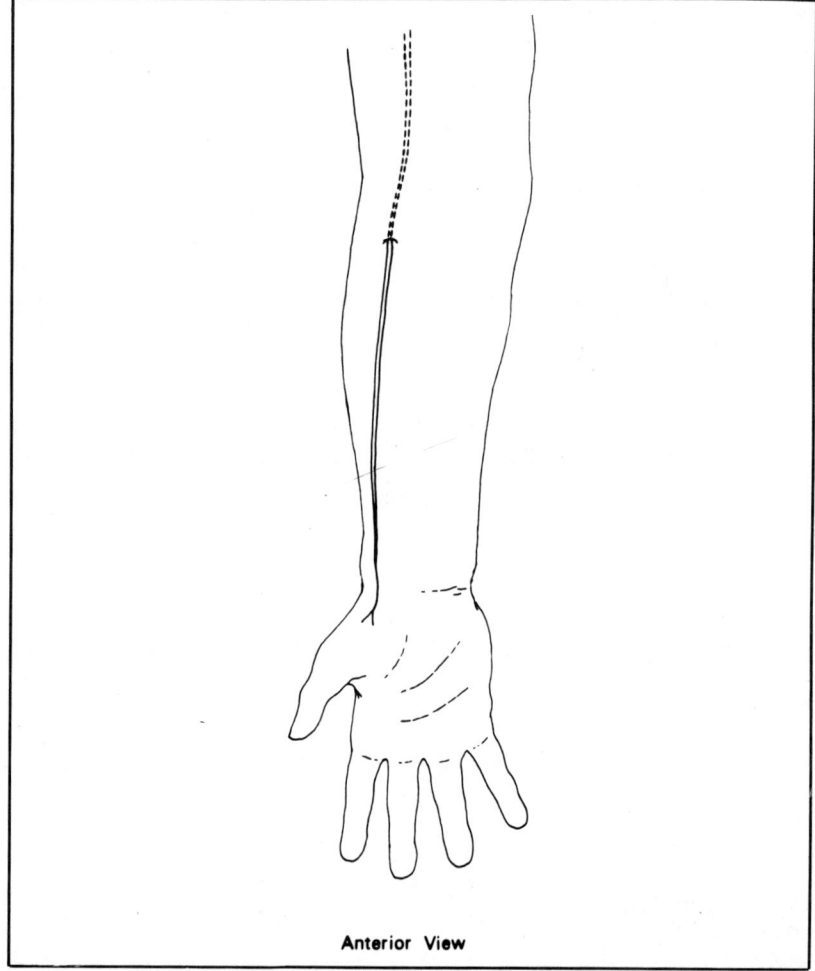

Figure 6-1
Superficial course of the lateral antebrachial cutaneous branch of the musculocutaneous nerve in the forearm.

Chapter 6 Musculocutaneous Nerve
(Sensory Studies)

ANATOMY

The *musculocutaneous nerve* receives fibers from $C_{5,6,7}$, which pass through the upper and middle trunks of the *brachial plexus* to the lateral cord. The musculocutaneous nerve is formed as one of two terminal branches of the lateral cord. It serves as the motor nerve to the coracobrachialis, biceps, and brachialis and supplies the skin over the radial aspect of the forearm as the *lateral (antebrachial) cutaneous nerve*, which descends along the anterolateral border of the forearm to the wrist (Fig. 6-1). The sensory fibers studied as described below originate from the C_6 root and travel via the upper trunk and lateral cord of the brachial plexus.

APPLICATIONS

Study results are useful in analyzing isolated lesions of the musculocutaneous nerve and aid in distinguishing C_6 radiculopathies from lesions of the upper trunk of the brachial plexus. Sensory responses may be obtainable in severe peripheral polyneuropathies after it is no longer possible to receive ulnar and median sensory responses [1].

PROCEDURE (SENSORY; ANTIDROMIC)

1. Place the cathode of the stimulating electrode in the elbow crease immediately lateral to the biceps tendon in such a way that the anode, cathode, and palpable radial pulse at the wrist are along a straight line (Fig. 6-2).

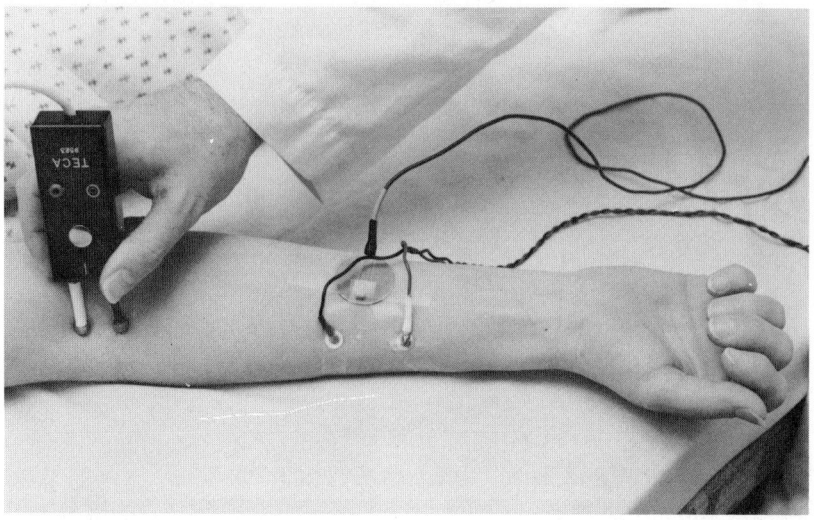

Figure 6-2
Electrode placement for antidromic sensory stimulation of the lateral antebrachial cutaneous branch of the musculocutaneous nerve.

2. The G_1 recording electrode is placed along the imaginary line, 12 cm distal to the cathode.
3. The G_2 electrode is similarly placed 3 cm distal to G_1.
4. Place the ground between G_1 and G_2.

NORMAL VALUES

Amplitude (μV)	Sensory Latency (msec)	Reference
> 12 (mean 24 ± 7.2)	< 2.6 (mean 2.3 ± 0.1)	[1]

REFERENCE

1. Lambert, E. H., and Daube, J. R. (Chairmen). *Special Course #16: Clinical Electromyography.* American Academy of Neurology Meeting, Chicago, Ill., April 23–28, 1979.

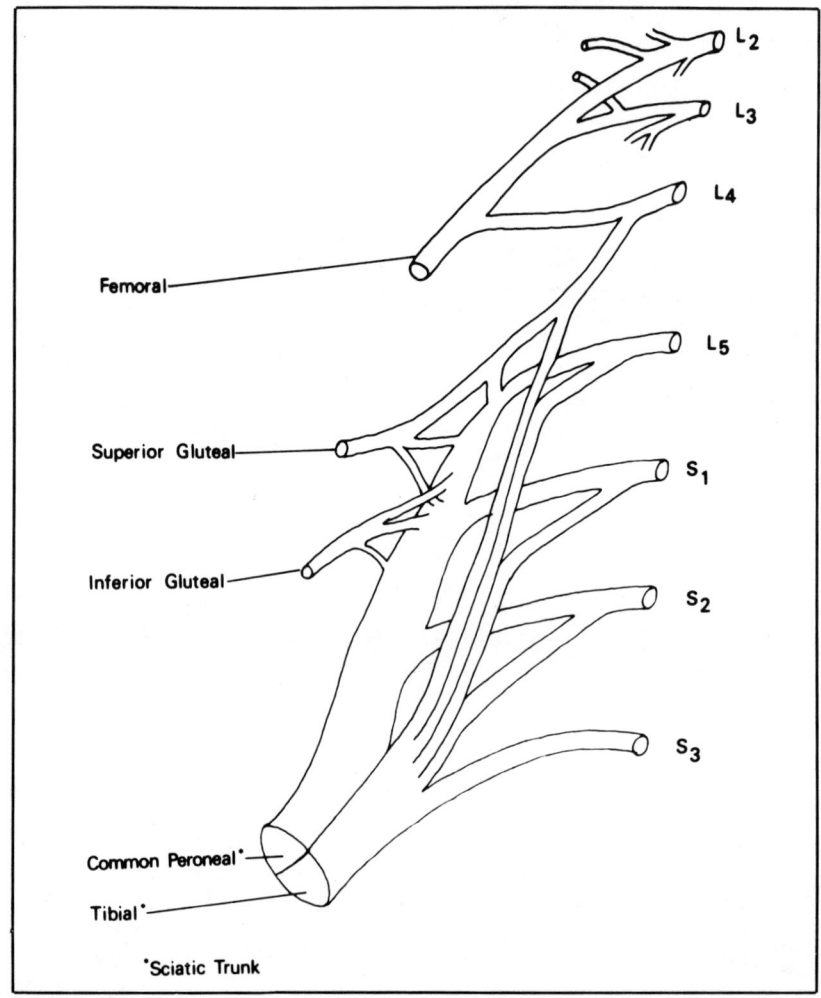

Figure 7-1
Simplified plan of the lumbosacral plexus emphasizing commonly studied nerves.

Chapter 7 Sciatic Nerve
(Motor Studies)

ANATOMY

The *spinal nerves* arise from the spinal cord within the spinal canal and pass out through the intervertebral foramina formed by the juxtaposition of the vertebral notches. Each spinal nerve is attached to the spinal cord by two roots: a ventral motor root and a dorsal sensory root. The motor and sensory roots merge immediately beyond the spinal ganglion to emerge through the intervertebral foramen as a spinal nerve. In the lumbosacral region the spinal nerves exit inferiorly to the vertebra of the same number. For example, spinal nerve L_4 exits between vertebrae L_4 and L_5. The spinal nerve then immediately splits into its two primary divisions; both dorsal and ventral primary divisions receive fibers from both roots. The dorsal primary divisions supply the muscles and skin of the dorsal part of the neck and trunk. The ventral primary divisions of the spinal nerves supply the ventral and lateral parts of the trunk and all parts of the limbs. The *lumbosacral plexus* (Fig. 7-1) consists of the combination of all the ventral primary divisions of the lumbar, sacral, and coccygeal nerves.

Fibers of the *sciatic nerve* originate from the ventral (anterior) primary divisions (rami) of the fourth and fifth lumbar spinal nerves and the first, second, and third sacral spinal nerves. These rami enter the *lumbosacral plexus* and emerge reorganized as the sciatic nerve, which exits from the pelvis through the greater sciatic notch. The sciatic nerve is actually two nerves within a common sheath: the *common peroneal* and the *tibial (posterior tibial) nerves*.

In the gluteal region, covered by the gluteus maximus muscle, the sciatic nerve runs laterally and downward to a point midway between

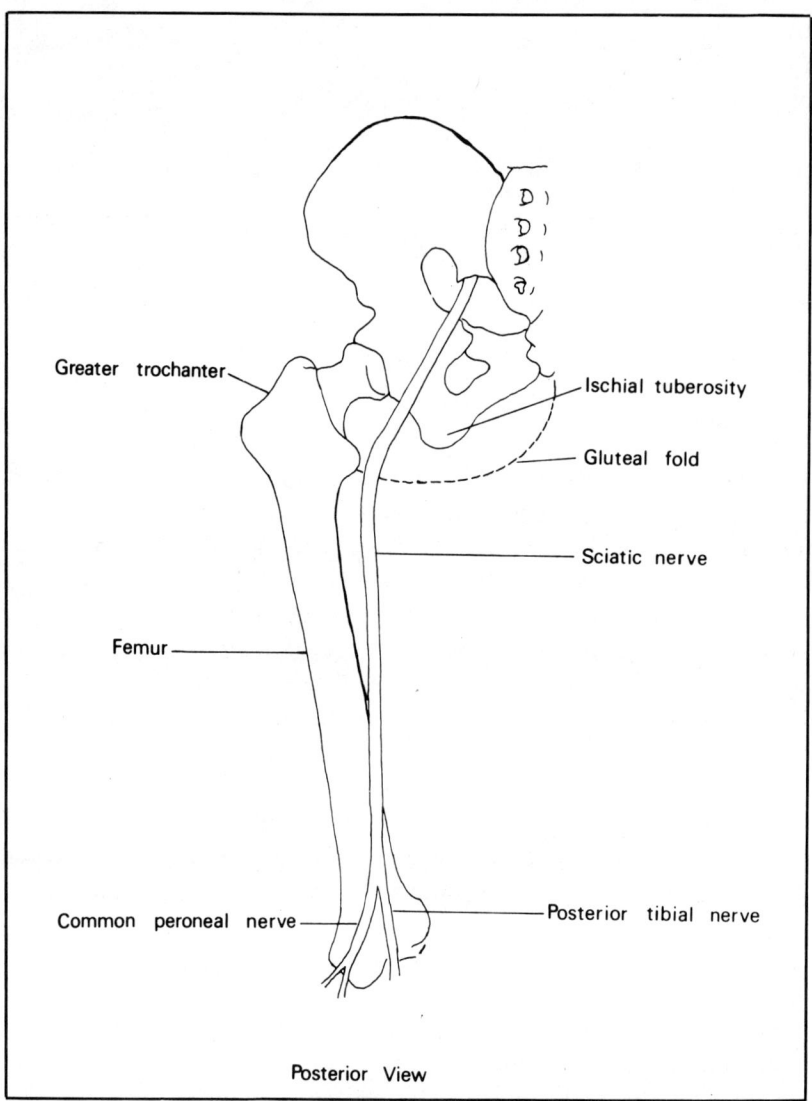

Figure 7-2
Landmarks for locating the superficial portion of the sciatic nerve trunk.

the ischial tuberosity and the greater trochanter of the femur. At the inferior margin of the buttock it occupies a superficial position in the angle between the gluteus maximus and the long head of the biceps femoris, at which point it is accessible to transcutaneous stimulation (Fig. 7-2).

The sciatic nerve trunk then enters the thigh, and at a variable distance above the popliteal fossa it divides into the common peroneal and tibial nerves. Fibers from the sciatic nerve convey cutaneous sensation from the lateral and posterior portions of the leg and the dorsal and plantar surfaces of the foot; sciatic nerve fibers also provide motor innervation to the hamstring muscles, a portion of the adductor magnus, and all the muscles of the leg and foot. Nerves to the semitendinosus, semimembranosus, biceps femoris, and adductor magnus are direct branches of the sciatic trunk before it bifurcates into the common peroneal and tibial nerves.

APPLICATIONS

Complete or partial "sciatic" palsy may be caused by lesions of the ventral nerve roots, the cauda equina, lumbosacral plexus, sciatic nerve trunk, the common peroneal nerve, or tibial nerve. A complete sciatic transection will cause a flail leg and foot. Combined with common peroneal and tibial nerve studies, assessment of the conduction velocities in the sciatic trunk may be helpful in localizing the lesion.

PROCEDURE

1. Electrode placement (Fig. 7-3)
    a. G_1 over the abductor digiti quinti.
    b. G_2 over the fifth toe.
    c. Ground between G_1 and G_2 on the dorsum of the foot.
2. Stimulation
    a. Transcutaneously, insert the cathode (50–70 mm monopolar EMG needle) in the gluteal skin fold equidistant between the ischial tuberosity and the greater trochanter of the femur. The disc anode must be placed nearby (Fig. 7-4).
    b. Percutaneously, place the cathode at the superior angle of the quadrangular popliteal space at the level of the upper border of the femoral condyles (Fig. 7-5).

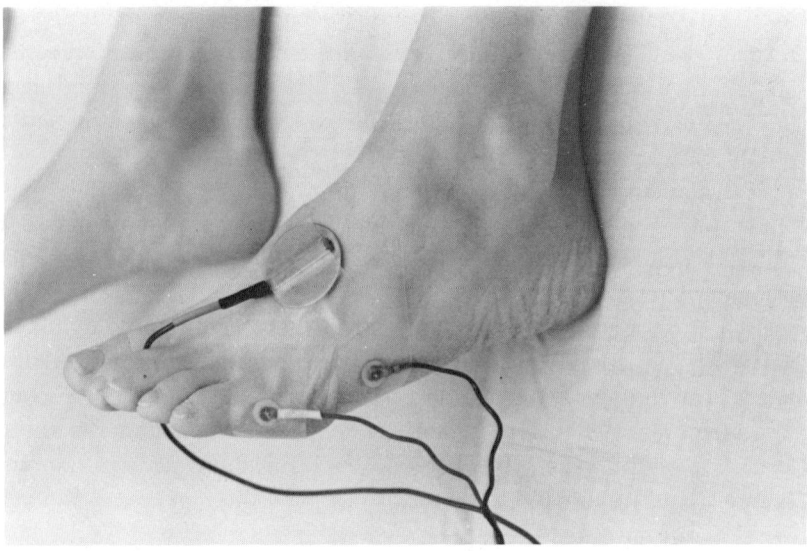

Figure 7-3
Recording electrode placement for recording from the abductor digiti quinti (lateral plantar branch of the posterior tibial nerve) in sciatic nerve conduction studies.

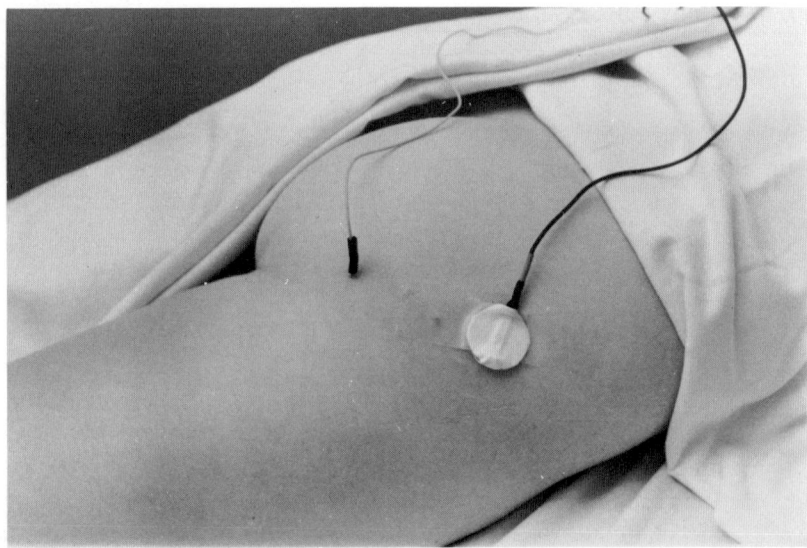

Figure 7-4
Stimulation of the sciatic nerve at the gluteal fold.

7. Sciatic Nerve

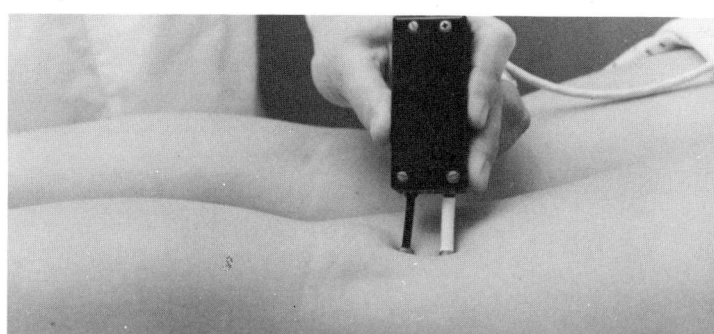

Figure 7-5
Stimulation of the posterior tibial branch of the sciatic nerve at the apex of the popliteal fossa.

NORMAL VALUES

Segment	NCV (m/sec)	Amplitude (mV)	Reference
Gluteal fold to popliteal fossa	51.3 ± 4.4 (45.3–61.1)	3–5	[1]

REFERENCE

1. Yap, C. B., and Hirota, T. Sciatic nerve motor conduction velocity study. *J. Neurol. Neurosurg. Psychiatry* 30:233, 1967.

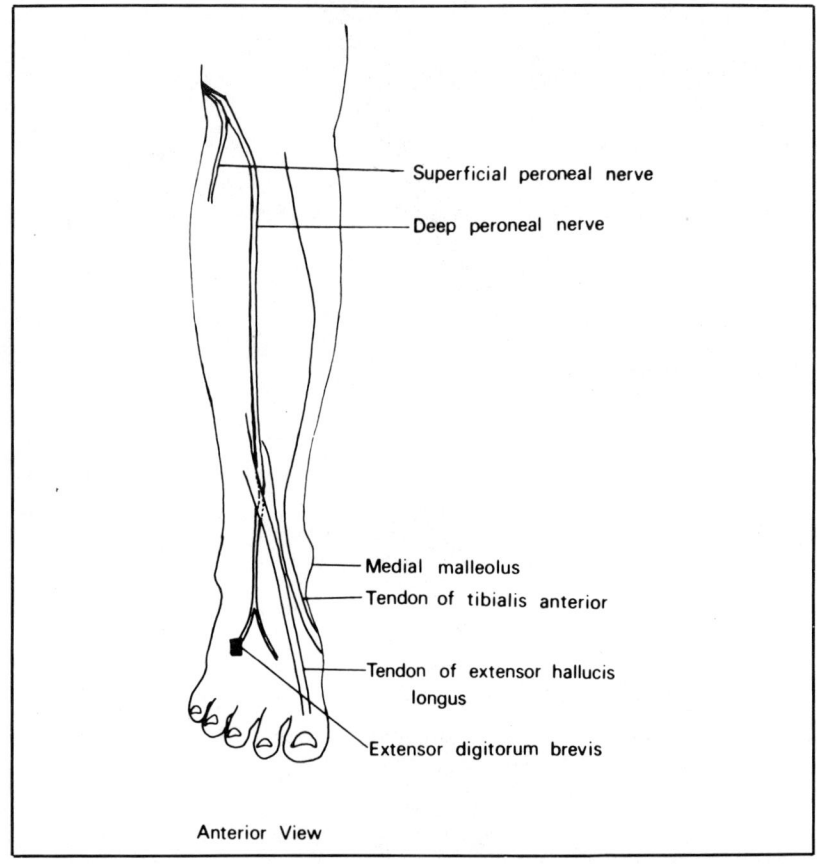

Figure 8-1
Motor branches of the common peroneal nerve.

Chapter 8 Peroneal Nerve
(Motor Studies)

ANATOMY

The *common peroneal nerve* and the *tibial nerve* are the two terminal divisions of the *sciatic nerve*. The common peroneal nerve is composed of fibers from L_4, L_5, S_1, and S_2. It runs laterally in the popliteal fossa, close to the medial border of the biceps femoris. It travels to the neck of the fibula, around which it winds, and then divides into the *superficial* and *deep peroneal nerves*. The deep peroneal nerve joins the anterior tibial artery in the proximal leg and then parallels this artery, passing under the extensor retinaculum and dividing into terminal medial and lateral branches at the ankle. The lateral terminal branch supplies the extensor digitorum brevis muscle; more proximal branches innervate the extensor muscles of the foot and toes. The peroneus longus and peroneus brevis are innervated by branches of the superficial peroneal nerve (Fig. 8-1).

APPLICATIONS

The common peroneal nerve is vulnerable to compression where it becomes superficial over the lateral aspect of the neck of the fibula. Injury to the peroneal nerve at this level causes impaired dorsiflexion and eversion of the foot and may also cause pain or paresthesias along the lateral surface of the leg, although the sensory fibers are less vulnerable to damage. In compression palsy of the common peroneal nerve, slowing may be present only in the segment across the head of the fibula. Therefore, a conduction velocity measured from the popliteal fossa to the ankle may fall within the normal range. To diagnose localized compression, the conduction velocity across the head of the

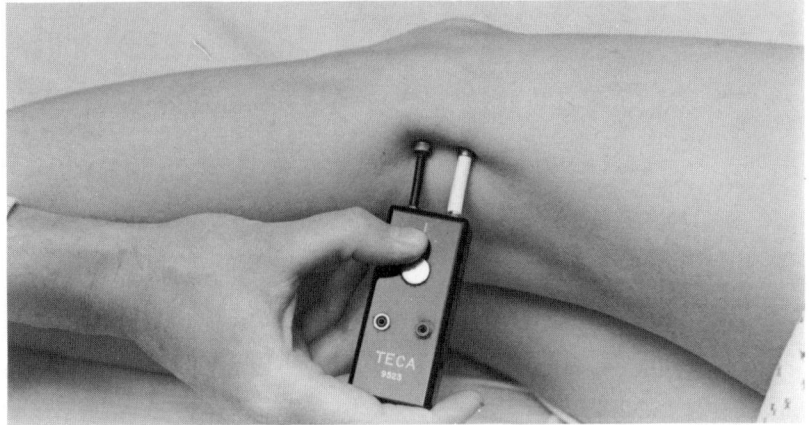

Figure 8-2
Stimulation of the common peroneal nerve in the popliteal fossa.

fibula should be more than 10 m per second slower than values recorded distal to the fibula. The common peroneal nerve is also often involved in generalized neuropathies such as those caused by uremia and diabetes mellitus.

PROCEDURE

1. Electrode placement (see Fig. 8-4)
   a. G_1 recording electrode over the extensor digitorum brevis muscle (EDB).
   b. G_2 recording electrode over the fifth toe.
   c. Ground over the dorsum of the foot between G_1 and G_2.
2. Stimulation
   a. Lateral aspect of the popliteal fossa just medial to the insertion of the tendon of the biceps femoris (Fig. 8-2).
   b. Along the anterolateral surface of fibula, 3 to 4 cm distal to the proximal tip of the fibular head (Fig. 8-3).
   c. Dorsal aspect of distal lower leg approximately 4 to 6 cm proximal to the medial malleolus and just medial to the tendon of the extensor hallucis muscle. This point is between the tendons of the tibialis anterior and the extensor hallucis proprius (Fig. 8-4). In about 20 percent of the population, the supply to the extensor digitorum brevis is by way of an accessory deep peroneal nerve which may be stimulated behind the lateral malleolus.

8. Peroneal Nerve

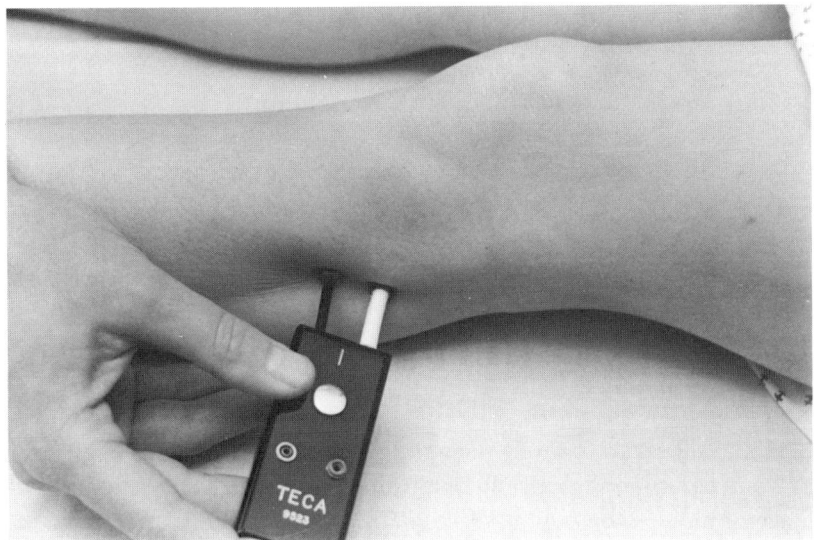

Figure 8-3
Stimulation of the deep peroneal nerve just distal to the fibular head.

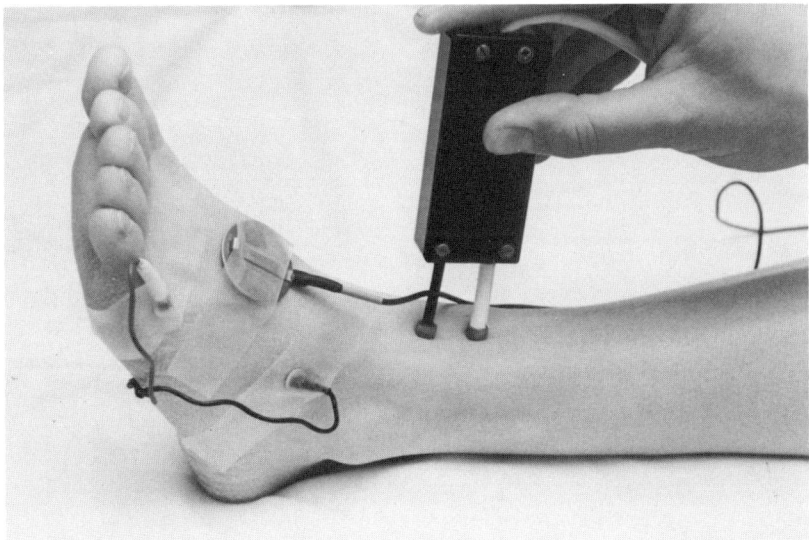

Figure 8-4
Electrode placement for recording from the extensor digitorum brevis and distal stimulation of the deep peroneal nerve.

NORMAL VALUES

Segment	Distal Latency or NCV	Amplitude (mV)	Reference
Ankle to EDB	5.1 msec	8.8 (6–12)	[1, 2]
Proximal to head of fibula to ankle	50 (SD 3.5) m/sec	8.8 (6–12)	[1, 2]
Distal to head of fibula to ankle	50 (SD 3.5) m/sec	8.8 (6–12)	[1, 2]

REFERENCES

1. Hodes, R., Larrabee, M. G., and German, W. The human electromyogram in response to nerve stimulation and conduction velocity of motor axons. *Arch. Neurol. Psychiatry* 60:340, 1948.
2. Lamontagne, A., and Buchthal, F. Electrophysiological studies in diabetic neuropathy. *J. Neurol. Neurosurg. Psychiatry* 33:442, 1970.

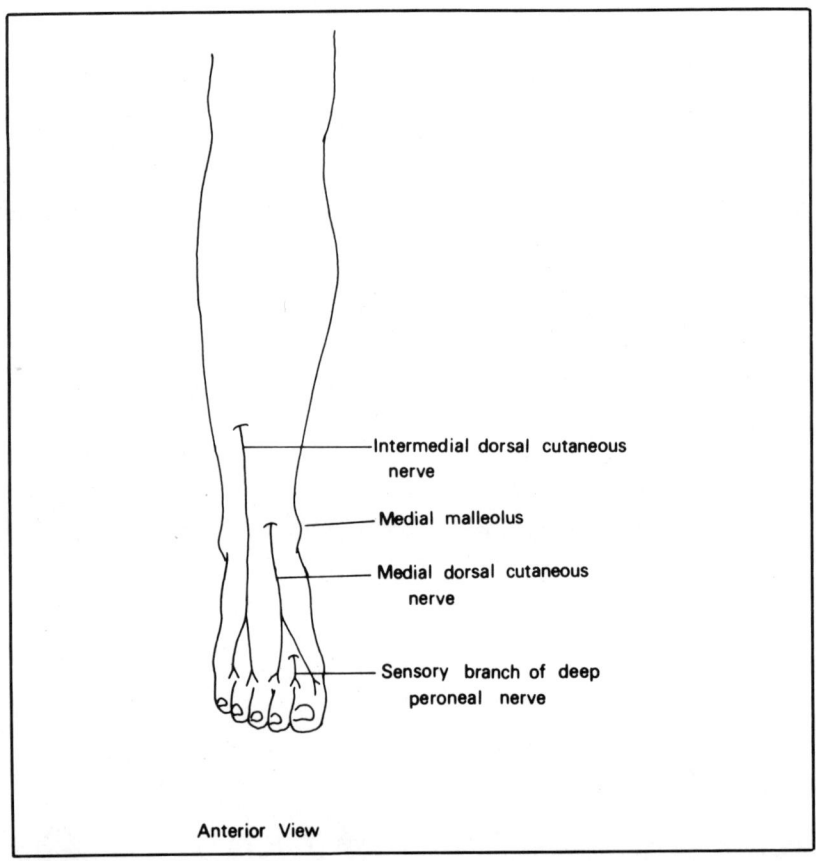

Figure 9-1
The distal sensory branches of the superficial peroneal nerve.

Chapter 9 Superficial Peroneal Nerve
(Sensory Studies)

ANATOMY

The *superficial peroneal nerve* receives its sensory fibers from the L_5 root segment, and, to a lesser extent, from the S_1 root segment. These fibers pass through the dorsal portion of the *sacral plexus* and travel distally with the common peroneal component of the *sciatic nerve*, the *common peroneal nerve*, and finally with the *superficial branch of the peroneal nerve*. The superficial peroneal nerve separates from the common peroneal nerve just distal to the fibular head, passes distally, and pierces the deep fascia in the lower third of the leg, soon dividing into the *medial* and *intermediate (intermedial) dorsal cutaneous nerves*, which supply sensation to the dorsum of the foot and toes (Fig. 9-1). The peroneus longus and peroneus brevis receive their motor innervation from proximal branches of the superficial peroneal nerve.

APPLICATIONS

Study of the superficial peroneal nerve is useful in distinguishing L_5 radiculopathies from more distal lesions. Values may become abnormal while the sural studies are still normal in developing polyneuropathies.

PROCEDURE (SENSORY; ANTIDROMIC)

1. Plantar-flex and invert the foot and palpate the superficial peroneal nerve (intermediate dorsal cutaneous branch) over the dorsum of the foot medial to the lateral malleolus (Fig. 9-1).
2. Place the G_1 recording electrode directly over the nerve 8 to 10 cm

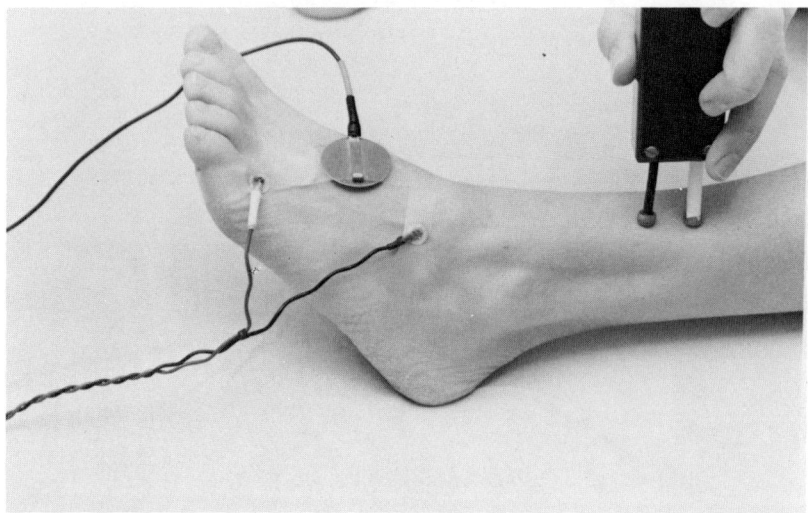

Figure 9-2
Electrode placement for antidromic stimulation of the intermedial dorsal cutaneous branch of the superficial peroneal nerve.

proximal to the most lateral interdigital web (Fig. 9-2).
3. Place the G_2 recording electrode 6 to 8 cm distal to the G_1 electrode near the base of the fifth toe.
4. Stimulate 10 cm proximal to the G_1 electrode along the anterolateral surface of the distal leg.

NORMAL VALUES

Age (years)	Latency (msec)	Amplitude (μV)	References
15	< 3.4 (mean 2.8)	> 5 (mean 14)	[1]
65	< 3.7 (mean 3.3)	> 5 (mean 6)	[1]

REFERENCE

1. Lambert, E. H., and Daube, J. R. (Chairmen). *Special Course #16: Clinical Electromyography.* American Academy of Neurology Meeting, Chicago, Ill., April 23–28, 1979.

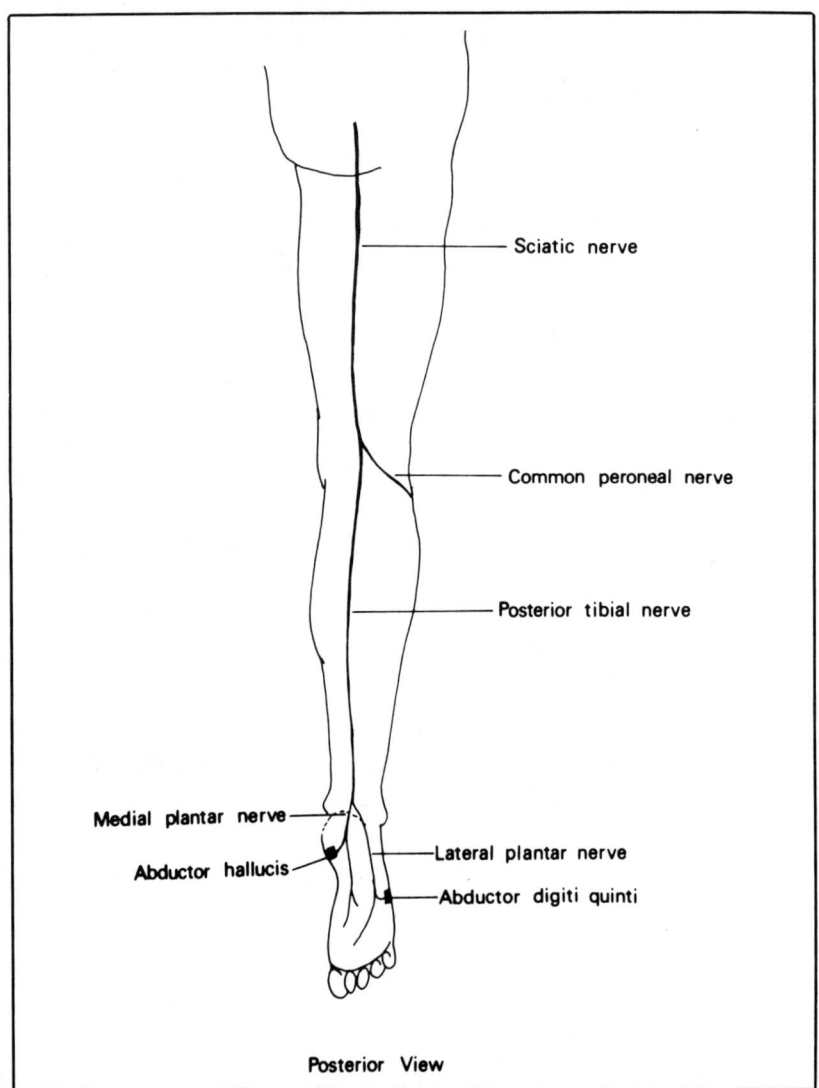

Figure 10-1
Origin and course of the posterior tibial nerve.

Chapter 10 Tibial Nerve
(Motor Studies)

ANATOMY

The *tibial nerve* (posterior tibial nerve) is composed of fibers from L_4, L_5, S_1, S_2, and S_3. It is the longer of the two medial branches formed by the bifurcation of the *sciatic nerve* at the upper corner of the quadrangular popliteal space. This nerve crosses the popliteal space, runs deep to the gastrocnemius and soleus muscles, and travels under the flexor retinaculum (tarsal tunnel) behind and inferior to the medial malleolus. At the distal end of the tarsal tunnel it bifurcates into the *medial* and *lateral plantar nerves*. The medial branch sends motor branches to the abductor hallucis and the lateral branch innervates the abductor digiti quinti (Fig. 10-1). The general distribution of the tibial nerve is to the posterior compartment muscles of the calf, the muscles and joints of the foot, and the skin of the heel and sole.

APPLICATIONS

The tibial nerve may be compromised in the popliteal space (e.g., by a popliteal aneurysm) or more distally at the ankle (tarsal tunnel syndrome). In the tarsal tunnel the trunk of the tibial nerve may be compromised or either of its two branches may be affected separately.

PROCEDURE

1. Electrode placement
   a. There are two alternatives:
      (1) G_1 recording electrode over the abductor hallucis to test the medial plantar branch (Fig. 10-2)

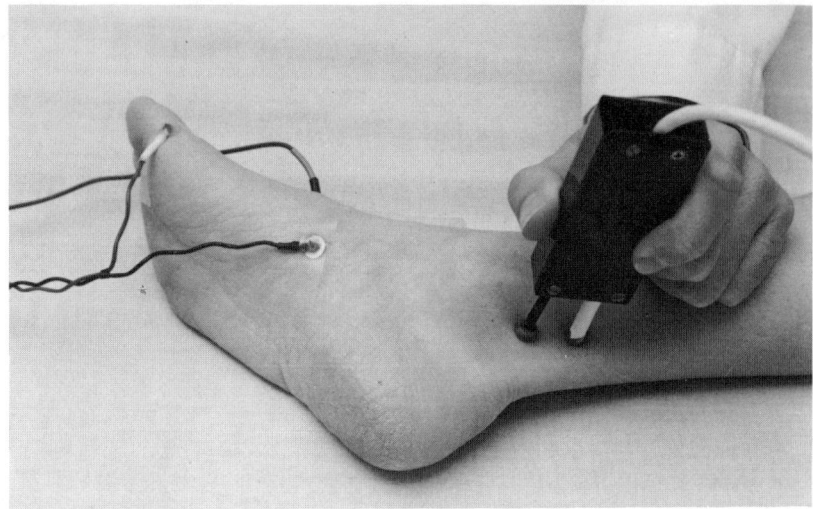

Figure 10-2
Electrode placement for recording from the abductor hallucis (medial plantar branch of the posterior tibial nerve) and point of distal stimulation for both medial and lateral plantar branches of the posterior tibial nerve.

      (2) G_1 recording electrode over the abductor digiti quinti to test the lateral plantar branch (Fig. 7-3).
  b. G_2 recording electrode over the great toe for method a(1) or over the fifth toe for method a(2).
  c. Ground between G_1 and G_2.
2. Stimulation
  a. Middle of the quadrangular popliteal space (Fig. 7-5).
  b. Slightly behind (posterior) and proximal to the medial malleolus (Fig. 10-2). Both plantar branches are stimulated at this point.

10. Tibial Nerve

NORMAL VALUES

Segment	Distal Latency or NCV	Amplitude (mV)	Reference
Above malleolus to abductor hallucis	≤ 6.1 msec	15.4 (8–22)	[1, 2]
Above malleolus to abductor digiti quinti	≤ 6.7 msec	15.4 (8–22)	[1, 2]
Popliteal fossa to above malleolus	51.2 (43.4–59.5) m/sec	15.4 (8–22)	[1, 2]

REFERENCES

1. Hodes, R., Larrabee, M. G., and German, W. The human electromyogram in response to nerve stimulation and conduction velocity of motor axons. *Arch. Neurol. Psychiatry* 60:340, 1948.
2. Jimenez, J., Easton, J. K. M., and Redford, J. B. Conduction studies of anterior and posterior tibial nerves. *Arch. Phys. Med. Rehabil.* 51:164, 1970.

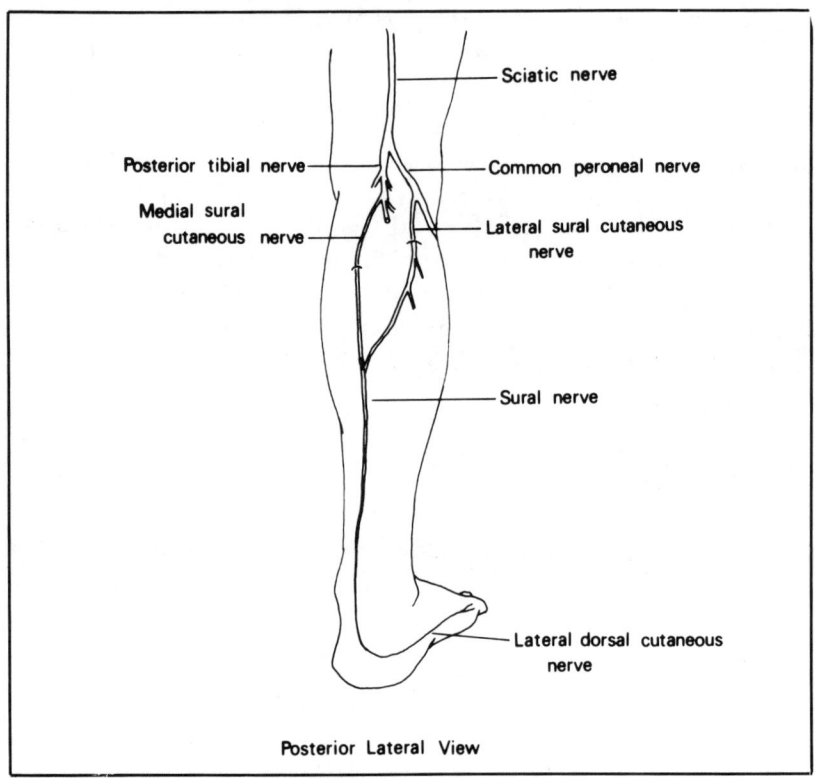

Figure 11-1
Origin and course of the sural nerve.

Chapter 11 Sural Nerve
(Sensory Studies)

ANATOMY

Sural sensory fibers originate from the S_1 root segment, traverse the *sacral plexus*, and course distally to the *sciatic nerve*. The *sural nerve* proper is formed by the union of the *medial sural cutaneous branch of the tibial nerve* and the *lateral sural cutaneous branch of the peroneal nerve*. The sural nerve becomes superficial at approximately midcalf after which it runs behind the lateral malleolus and becomes the *lateral dorsal cutaneous nerve* over the dorsum of the foot (Fig. 11-1). In patients with an accessory *deep peroneal nerve*, it may be necessary to perform testing of the sural nerve orthodromically because of the large muscle potential from the extensor digitorum brevis that results after stimulation in the midcalf.

APPLICATIONS

Study of the sural nerve is useful in distinguishing S_1 and S_2 radiculopathies from lesions involving and distal to the S_1 dorsal root ganglion. The sural nerve often develops abnormal responses—especially amplitude decrement—early in the course of polyneuropathies. It may be impossible to evoke an action potential from the sural nerve in persons more than sixty years old.

PROCEDURE (SENSORY; ANTIDROMIC)

1. Palpate the sural nerve behind (posterior-inferior to) the lateral malleolus.
2. Place the G_1 recording electrode over the sural nerve at the point of palpation (Fig. 11-2).

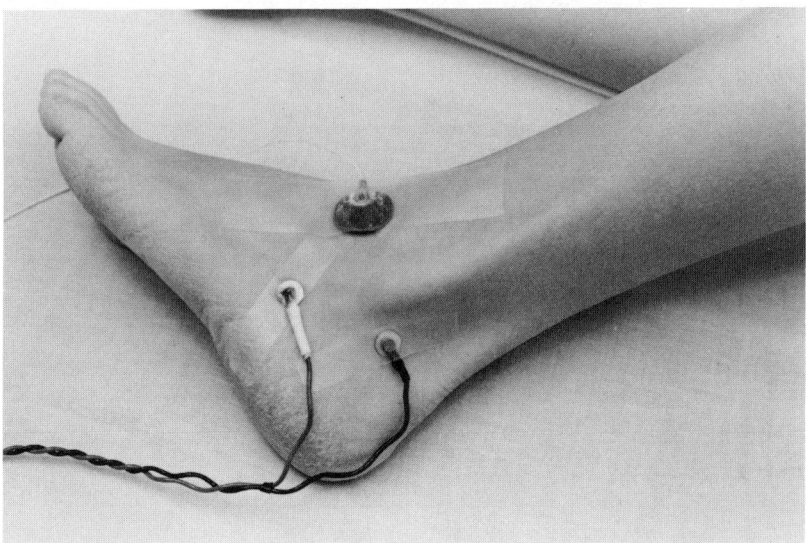

Figure 11-2
Recording electrode placement for the sural nerve.

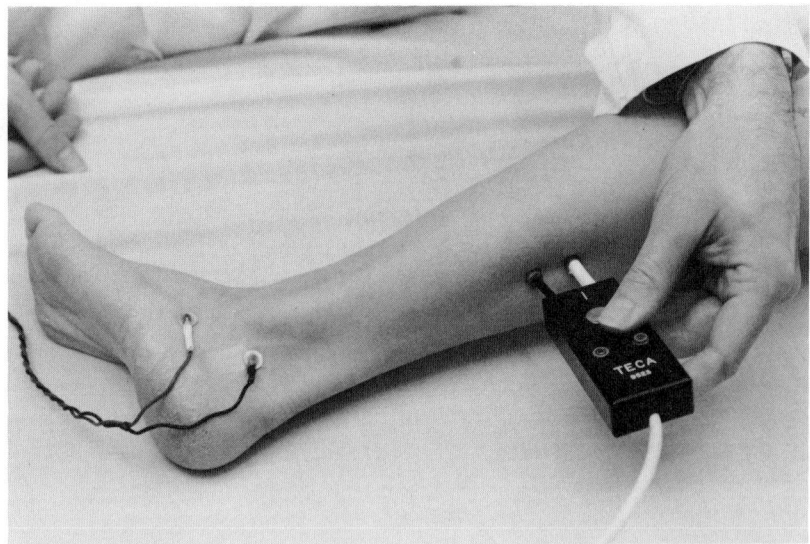

Figure 11-3
Antidromic stimulation of the sural nerve in midcalf.

11. Sural Nerve

3. Place the G_2 recording electrode 3 cm distal to the G_1 electrode along the course of the lateral dorsal cutaneous nerve.
4. Place the ground over the dorsum of the foot between G_1 and G_2.
5. Stimulate with the cathode located in the midcalf 14 cm proximal to the G_1 recording electrode (Fig. 11-3).

NORMAL VALUES

Age (years)	Amplitude (μV)	Latency (msec)	Reference
15	> 5 (mean 15)	< 4.2 (mean 3.6)	[1]
65	> 3 (mean 8)	< 4.6 (mean 3.9)	[1]

REFERENCE

1. Lambert, E. H., and Daube, J. R. (Chairmen). *Special Course #16: Clinical Electromyography.* American Academy of Neurology Meeting, Chicago, Ill., April 23–28, 1979.

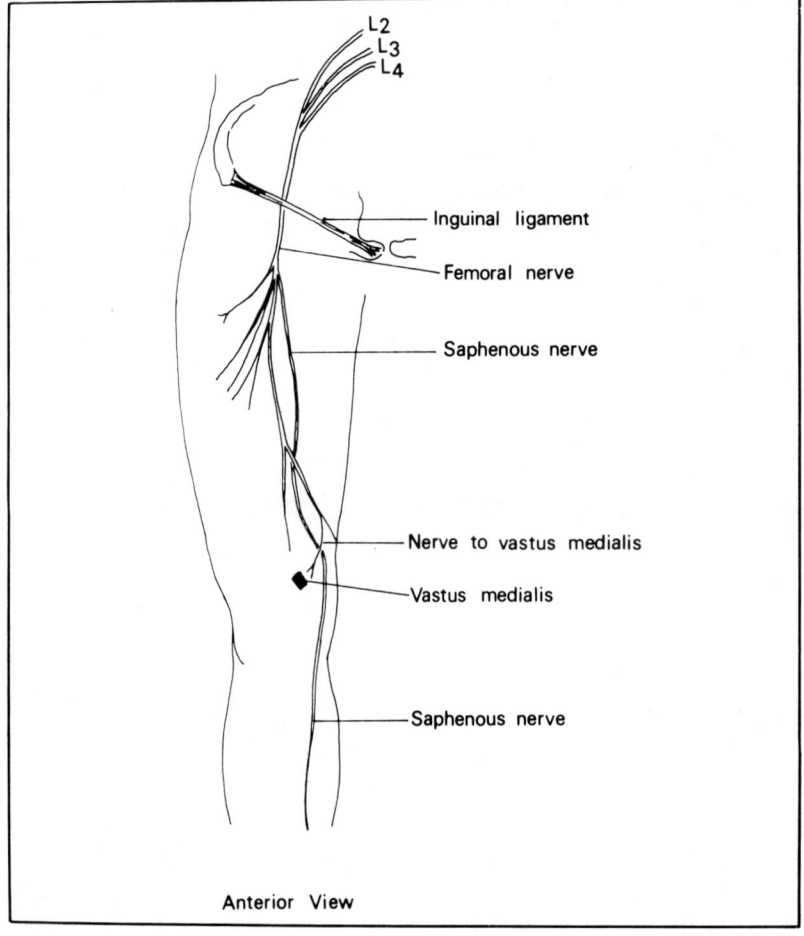

Figure 12-1
Origin and course of the femoral nerve.

Chapter 12 Femoral Nerve
(Motor Studies)

ANATOMY

Receiving fibers from $L_{2,3,4}$, the *femoral nerve* is the largest branch of the *lumbar plexus*. It passes through the psoas muscle and exits from the abdominal cavity under the inguinal ligament lateral to the femoral artery. Soon after entering the thigh, it breaks up into various branches, the largest and longest of which is the *saphenous nerve*. The femoral nerve supplies motor innervation to the iliacus, pectineus, sartorius, and quadriceps femoris as well as sensory innervation to the skin over the lateral and anterior aspects of the thigh (Fig. 12-1). The quadriceps femoris consists of the rectus femoris, vastus lateralis, vastus medialis, and vastus intermedius. The EMAP of the vastus medialis is generally used in motor conduction studies of the femoral nerve (Fig. 12-2).

APPLICATIONS

Femoral neuropathy may be caused by multiple systemic factors, notably diabetes mellitus and alcoholism. Compression or injury of the nerve has been reported with hemorrhage into the psoas muscle, pelvic fractures, increased intra-abdominal pressure during vaginal delivery, pressure by surgical retractor blades on the psoas muscle, and a prolonged dorsal lithotomy position during operations with compression at the level of the inguinal ligament [2].

PROCEDURE

1. Electrode placement (Fig. 12-5)

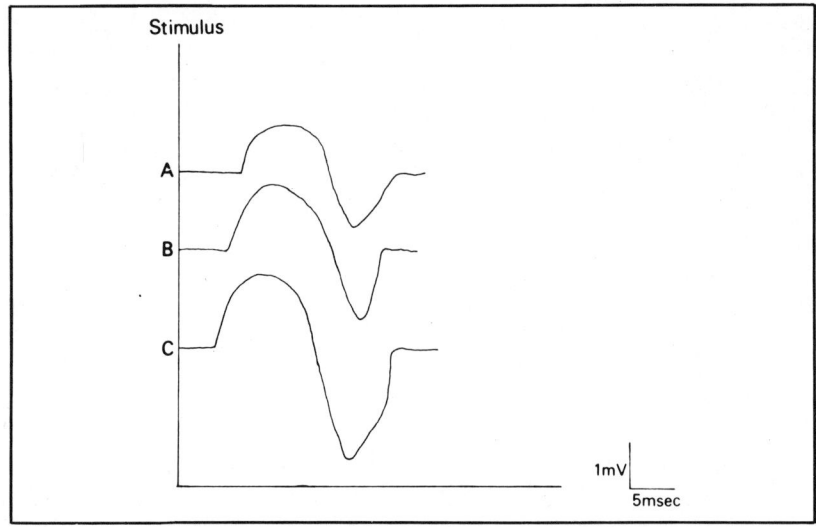

Figure 12-2
Evoked muscle action potentials from the vastus medialis from above the inguinal ligament (A), below the inguinal ligament (B), and at Hunter's canal (C).

    a. G_1 recording needle electrode near the motor point of the vastus medialis.
    b. G_2 recording electrode over the proximal tibia.
    c. Ground over the distal femur between G_1 and G_2.
2. Stimulation (percutaneous)
    a. Just proximal to the inguinal ligament over the projected course of the femoral nerve (Fig. 12-3).
    b. Just distal to the inguinal ligament, lateral to the palpable femoral artery in the femoral triangle (Fig. 12-4).
    c. At Hunter's canal along the medial aspect of the thigh. Hunter's canal is deep to the sartorius muscle along the middle third of the thigh (Figs. 12-5 and 12-6).
3. Stimulation (transcutaneous). Transcutaneous stimulation (EMG needle) can be used and seems to produce less discomfort, especially in obese or muscular patients. With transcutaneous stimulation, a low to moderate intensity is used while the needle is gradually advanced. As the needle tip approaches the femoral nerve, the vastus medialis can be observed to contract, thus making it possible to avoid insertion directly into the nerve [3]. The disc anode is placed over the anterior thigh well lateral to the femoral triangle. Transcutaneous stimulation is especially useful at Hunter's canal. Also, if

12. Femoral Nerve

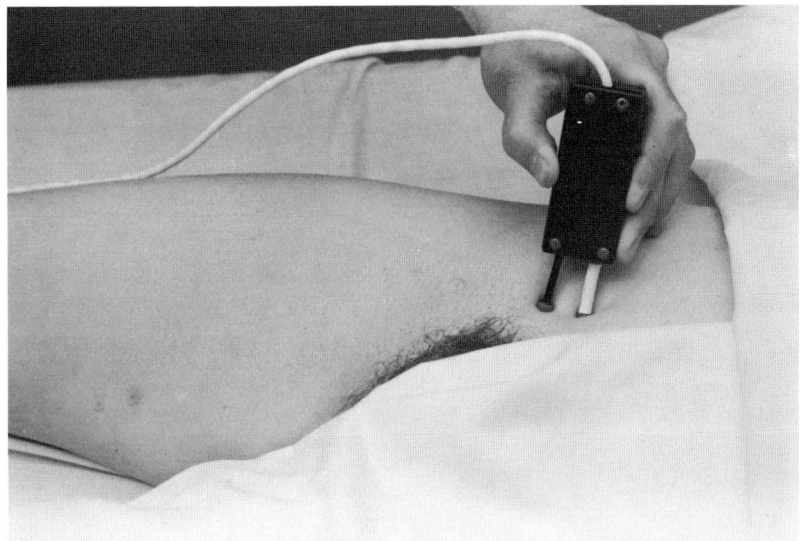

Figure 12-3
Stimulation of the femoral nerve proximal to the inguinal ligament.

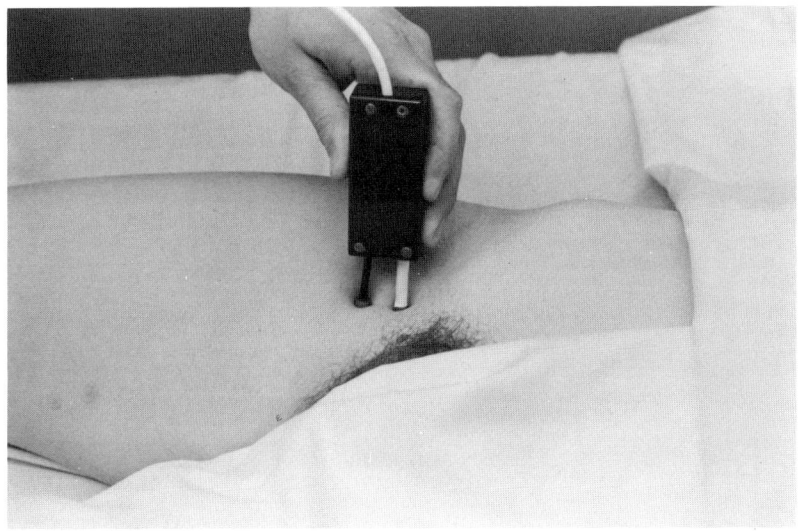

Figure 12-4
Stimulation of the femoral nerve distal to the inguinal ligament.

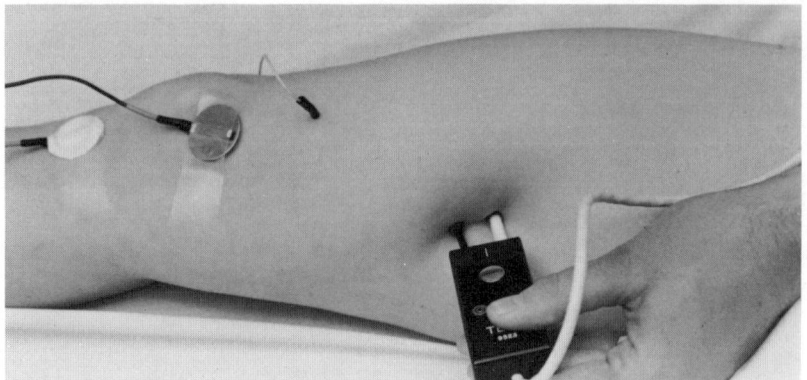

Figure 12-5
Electrode placement for recording from the vastus medialis and stimulation of the femoral nerve at Hunter's canal.

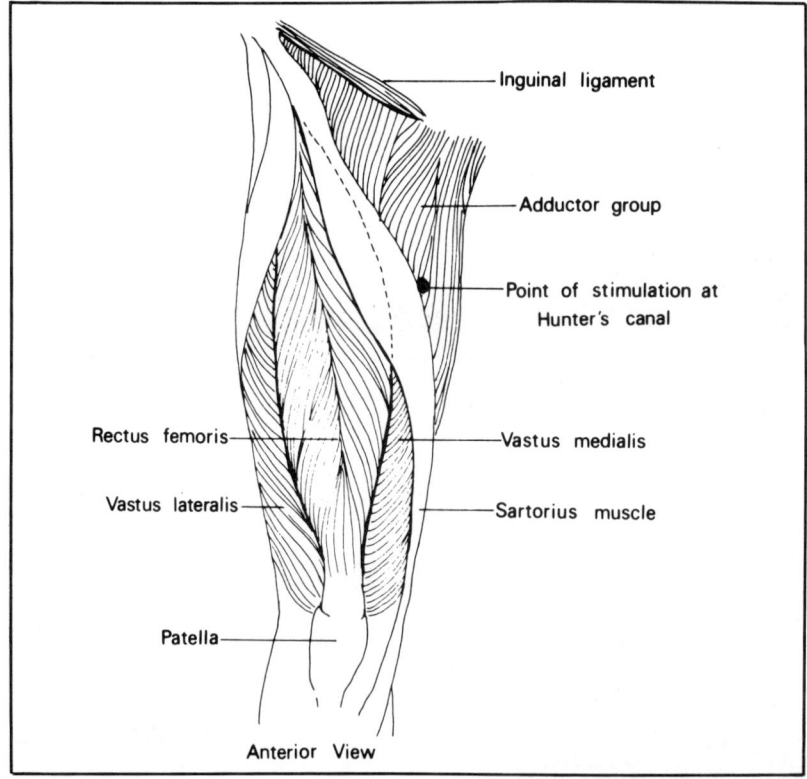

Figure 12-6
Location of the stimulation point at Hunter's canal.

latencies are unusually prolonged with percutaneous stimulation, one may be seeing an H-reflex rather than the desired M-response. Transcutaneous stimulation is useful in resolving this difficulty.

NORMAL VALUES

(Values taken from Johnson [1]).

	Mean	SD	Range
Distance from above inguinal ligament to vastus medialis	35.2 cm	1.9 cm	29–38 cm
Latency from above inguinal ligament to vastus medialis	7.1 msec	0.7 msec	6.1–8.4 msec
Latency from below inguinal ligament to vastus medialis	6.0 msec	0.7 msec	5.5–7.5 msec
Latency from Hunter's canal to vastus medialis	4.0 msec	...	...
NCV from above inguinal ligament to Hunter's canal	66.7 m/sec	7.4 m/sec	50–96 m/sec
NCV from below inguinal ligament to Hunter's canal	69.4 m/sec	9.2 m/sec	50–90 m/sec
Distance across inguinal ligament	5.5 cm	1.6 cm	4.2–6.6 cm

REFERENCES

1. Johnson, E. W., Wood, D. K., and Powers, J. J. Femoral nerve conduction studies. *Arch. Phys. Med. Rehabil.* 49:528, 1968.
2. Kopell, P., and Thompson, W. A. L. *Peripheral Entrapment Neuropathies.* Baltimore: Williams & Wilkins, 1963.
3. Lambert, E. H., and Daube, J. R. (Chairmen). *Special Course #16: Clinical Electromyography.* American Academy of Neurology Meeting, Chicago, Ill., April 23–28, 1979.

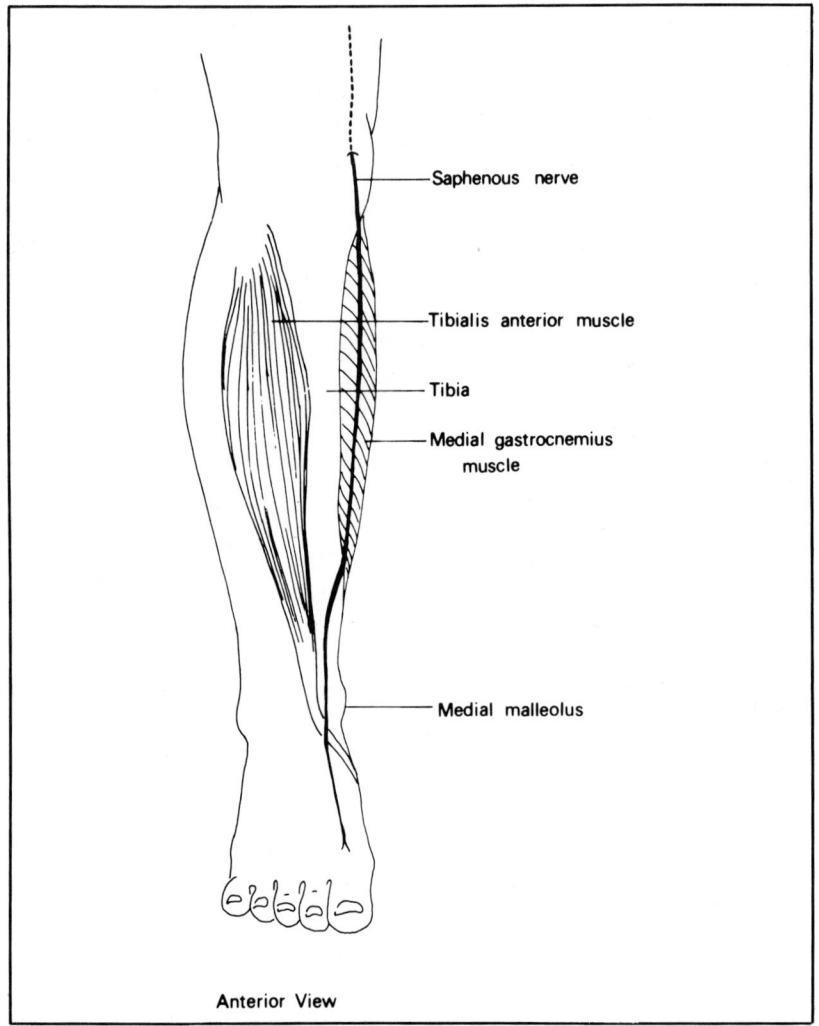

Figure 13-1
Distal superficial course of the saphenous nerve.

Chapter 13 Saphenous Nerve
(Sensory Studies)

ANATOMY

The *saphenous nerve* receives contributions from the L_3 and L_4 root segments which pass through the dorsal portion of the *lumbar plexus* before passing distally in the *femoral nerve*. The saphenous nerve is the largest and longest division of the femoral nerve, which branches just distal to the inguinal ligament. The saphenous nerve runs down the medial side of the thigh and leg, in front of the medial malleolus, and terminates on the dorsum of the foot at about the level of the first metatarsophalangeal joint (Fig. 13-1).

APPLICATIONS

Study of the saphenous nerve is useful in distinguishing L_3 and L_4 radiculopathies from lesions involving and distal to the L_3 and L_4 dorsal root ganglia.

PROCEDURE (SENSORY; ANTIDROMIC)

1. Place the G_2 recording electrode in the space between the highest prominence of the medial malleolus and the medial border of the tibialis anterior tendon (Fig. 13-2).
2. Place the G_1 recording electrode 3 cm proximal to the G_2 electrode along a line just medial and parallel to the tibialis anterior tendon.
3. Stimulate the saphenous nerve deep to the medial border of the tibia with the stimulating cathode located 14 cm proximal to the G_1 recording electrode. The stimulating electrodes must be pushed in firmly between the medial belly of the gastrocnemius and tibia; re-

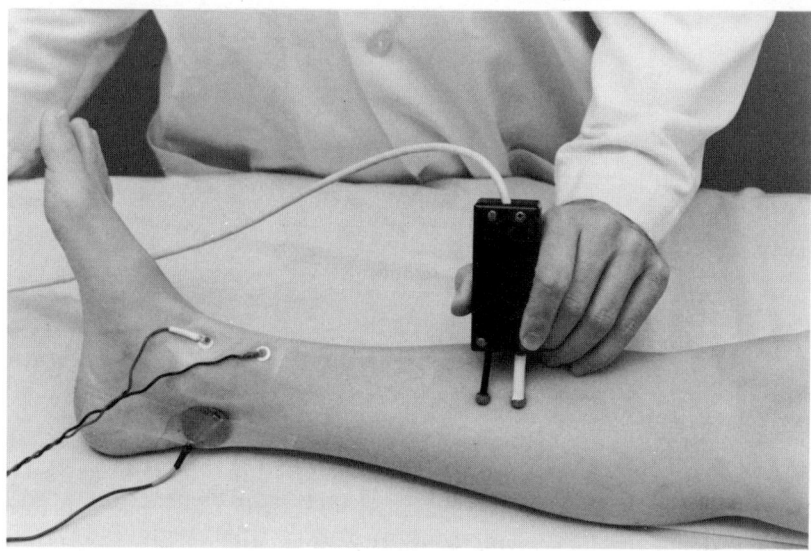

Figure 13-2
Electrode placement for antidromic stimulation of the saphenous nerve.

laxation of the gastrocnemius, achieved by slight plantar flexion of the foot at the ankle, is often helpful.

NORMAL VALUES

Latency (msec)	Amplitude (μV)	Reference
3.6 ± 0.4 SD	9 ± 3.4 SD ($\leq$ 5 in ⅓ of cases)	[1]

REFERENCE

1. Lambert, E. H., and Daube, J. R. (Chairmen). *Special Course #16: Clinical Electromyography.* American Academy of Neurology Meeting, Chicago, Ill., April 23–28, 1979.

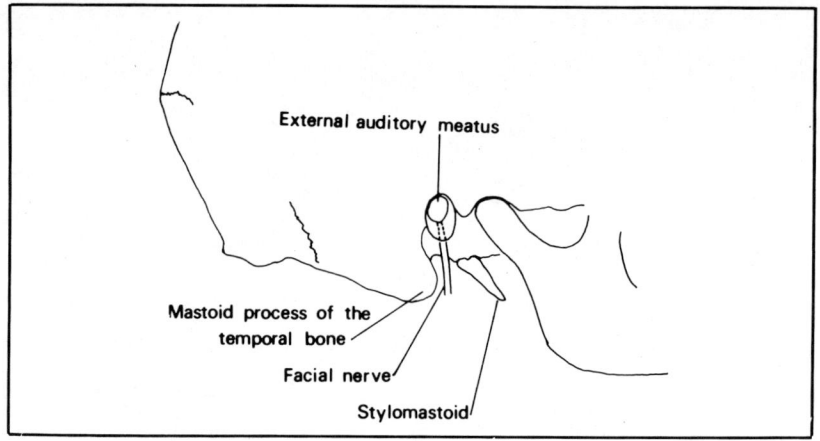

Figure 14-1
Facial nerve in relationship to the mastoid process of the temporal bone.

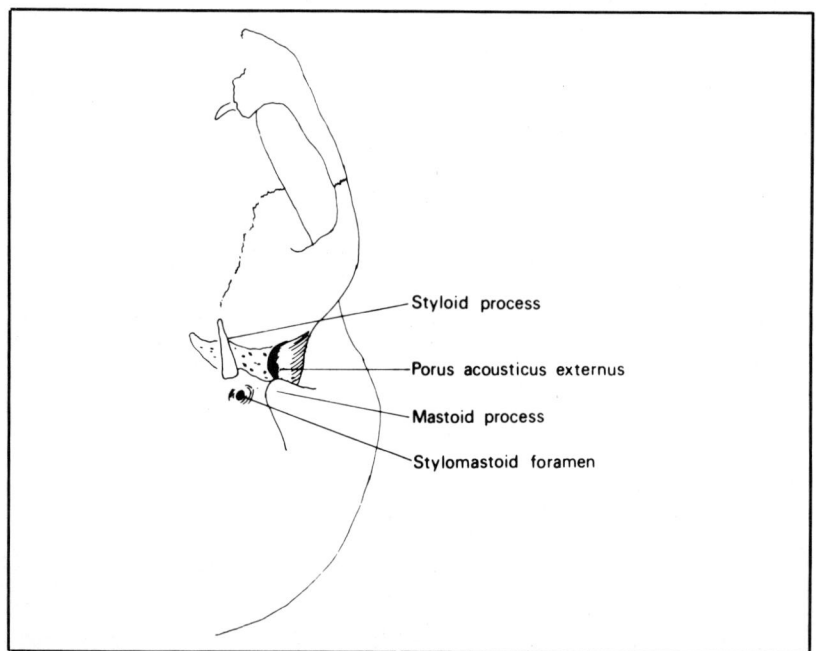

Figure 14-2
Stylomastoid foramen in relationship to the mastoid process of the temporal bone.

Chapter 14 Facial Nerve Stimulation
(Motor Studies)

ANATOMY

The motor division of the *seventh cranial nerve* contains special visceral efferent fibers which innervate the muscles of facial expression (mimetic muscles), the platysma, and the buccinator. These motor fibers emerge from the ventral aspect of the caudal pons and exit from the skull via the stylomastoid foramen (Figs. 14-1 and 14-2). The nerve then traverses the substance of the parotid gland behind the mandibular ramus, spreading out in an irregular series of branches ultimately supplying the orbicularis oculi, nasalis, buccinator, orbicularis oris, and platysma.

APPLICATIONS

At the present time there is no satisfactory electrodiagnostic method for predicting within the first day or two following onset of Bell's palsy which patients will subsequently develop complete loss of function of the facial nerve. However, nerve conduction studies done five to seven days after the onset of the paralysis are of prognostic significance [1]:

1. Normal results: complete recovery with only a very small chance of aberrant regeneration of the facial nerve.
2. Evoked response of reduced amplitude and prolonged latency: usually good recovery but some chance of aberrant regeneration with facial synkinesis or crocodile-tear phenomenon, or both.
3. No response: high incidence of aberrant regeneration; otherwise, most patients will have satisfactory recovery of function, but a few patients in this group may have no functional recovery.

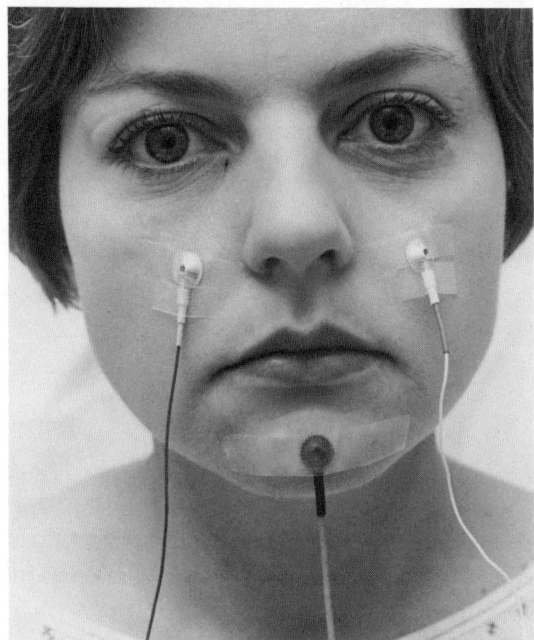

Figure 14-3
Recording electrode placement for right facial nerve stimulation. Note that the G_1 electrode has a black wire and is under the right eye.

The procedure described below concerns the nasalis muscle. Using different electrode placements, recordings can also be made from the mentalis, orbicularis oris, and orbicularis oculi.

PROCEDURE

1. Using silver or silver chloride discs, place the G_1 electrode over the nasalis muscle 1 cm above the external naris directly beneath the pupil. Needle electrodes can also be used for recording (Fig. 14-3).
2. Place the G_2 electrode in the same position on the opposite side of the face.
3. Place the ground on the chin.
4. Stimulate with a hand-held bipolar surface prong.
    a. Place the cathode near the stylomastoid foramen just below and anterior to the lower tip of the mastoid, beneath the earlobe. The anode should be inferior to the cathode and must often be rotated to reduce artifact or eliminate masseter contraction (Fig. 14-4).

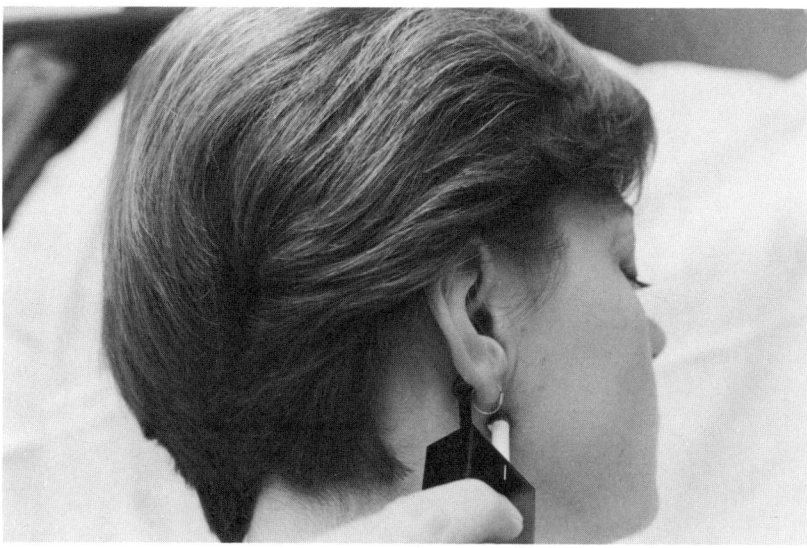

Figure 14-4
Facial nerve stimulation near the stylomastoid foramen.

  b. If method a fails, the cathode can be placed just anterior and inferior to the tragus of the earlobe (Fig. 14-5).
5. The initial deflection must be negative in order to measure the latency.

NORMAL VALUES

Values must always be compared with those from the opposite facial nerve; a difference in latencies of more than 0.6 msec represents a significant abnormality [1]. The distance from the cathode to the active recording electrode must be identical on the two sides. The amplitude is measured from the baseline to the negative peak. The latency is the time from the shock artifact to the initial negative deflection. The distance is from the cathode to the active recording electrode (G_1).

	Amplitude (mV)	Latency (msec)	Distance (cm)
Range	1.8–4.0	1.5–4.0	8–14
Mean	2.2	2.7	...

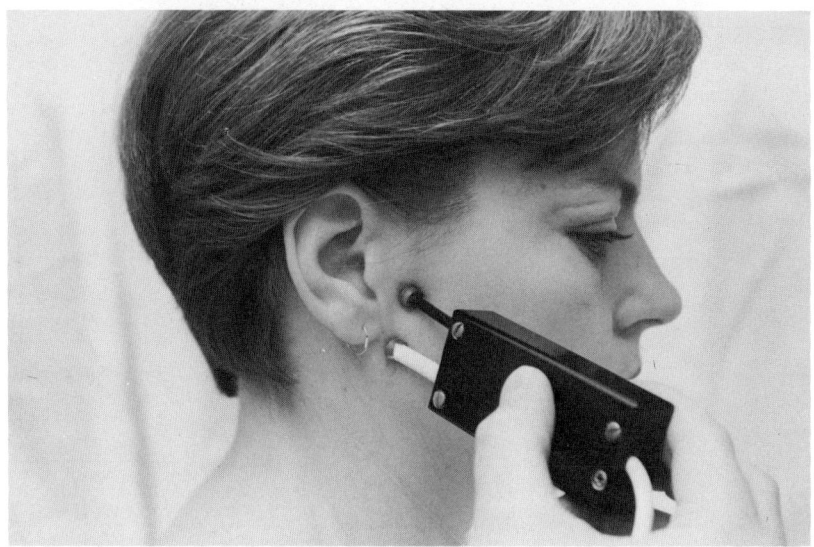

Figure 14-5
Facial nerve stimulation anterior and inferior to the tragus.

REFERENCE

1. Lambert, E. H., and Daube, J. R. (Chairmen). *Special Course #16: Clinical Electromyography.* American Academy of Neurology Meeting, Chicago, Ill., April 23–28, 1979.

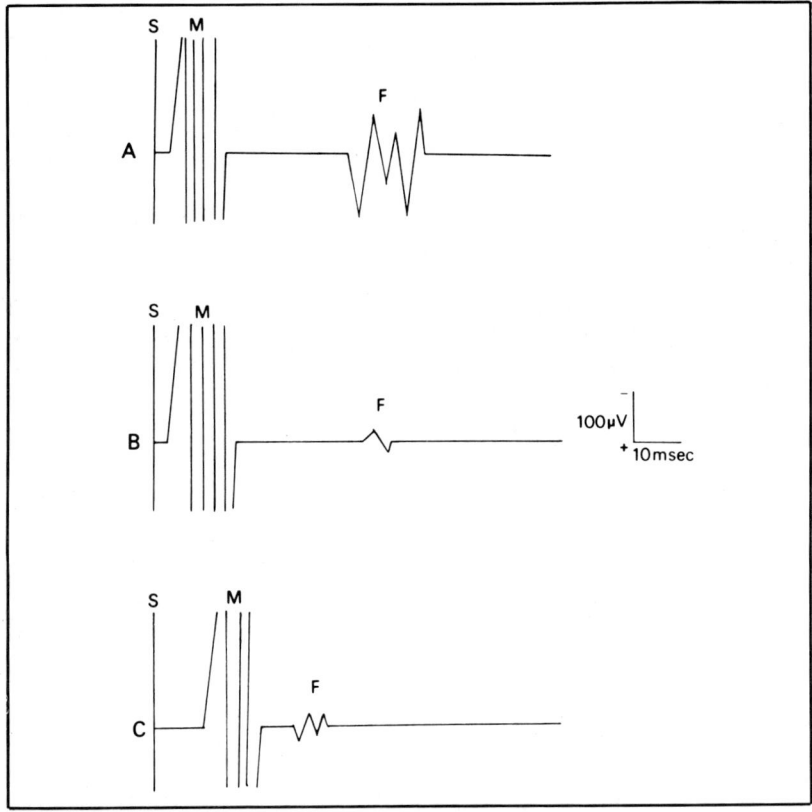

Figure 15-1
F-wave with distal (A and B) and proximal (C) stimulation of the same nerve. Note variation of latency, amplitude, and configuration in A and B; more proximal stimulation results in a shorter F-wave latency (C). Stimulus (S) and M-response (M) are off the vertical scale.

Chapter 15 The F-Wave

ANATOMY AND PHYSIOLOGY

F-waves are compound muscle action potentials recorded from the muscle fibers innervated by motor axons that probably have been activated by antidromic nerve action potentials ascending in motor axons to the anterior horn cells [3]. The latency of an F-wave includes the time required for the evoked action potential to ascend antidromically to the anterior horn cells and the time required for the resultant action potential to descend orthodromically from the anterior horn cell to the muscle fibers. The supramaximal stimulus typically used activates only a small percentage of the motor units, and F-wave responses vary in latency (by a few milliseconds), amplitude, and configuration from stimulus to stimulus. F-waves are of lower amplitude than the directly (orthodromically) evoked M-waves (Fig. 15-1). The latency *increases* with more distal sites of stimulation because the antidromic and orthodromic distances increase. The latency measure is taken from the onset of the earliest reproducible potential in the series of recorded F-waves. However, some investigators recommend using the average latency of 10 responses [1]. Stimulation of the ulnar, median, and tibial nerves evokes F-waves most reliably. Study of the F-wave response of the peroneal nerve is more difficult. The normal parameters of the F-wave are summarized below:

Threshold	Persists with supramaximal stimulation
Latency	Varies from stimulus to stimulus by a few milliseconds (increases with more distal sites of stimulation)

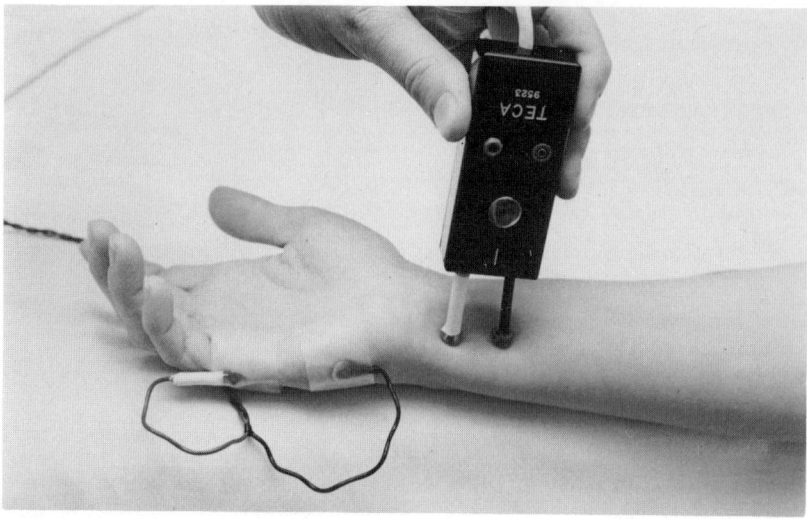

Figure 15-2
Electrode placement for F-wave determination with ulnar nerve stimulation. Note that the cathode is **proximal** *to the anode.*

Amplitude	Variable with each response; ranges from 50 to 300 μV
Configuration	Variable with each response; triphasic to polyphasic

APPLICATIONS

Measurement of F-wave latencies may be of value in identifying disorders involving proximal segments of peripheral nerves, plexuses, nerve roots, and the spinal cord, especially when these results are combined with routine motor and sensory conduction velocities and nerve root stimulation studies. The determination of F-wave latencies is thought to be particularly valuable in evaluating neuropathies in which focal, proximal pathology may be seen, as in Guillain-Barré syndrome and the neuropathy associated with rheumatoid arthritis [1].

PROCEDURE

1. Set gain voltage at 200 to 500 μV per centimeter.
2. Set the sweep speed at 5 msec per centimeter in the upper extremity and 10 msec per centimeter in the lower extremity.

3. With the cathode **proximal** to the anode, apply a supramaximal stimulus to the distal median, ulnar, or tibial nerves using the standard electrode placements (Fig. 15-2).
4. Stimulate more proximally to be certain the F-wave latency *shortens*.
5. Record 20 F-waves stimulating distally, and use the shortest reproducible (within a few milliseconds) latency.
6. With the arm in a 90-degree angle of abduction, measure the arm distance from the cathode to the sternoclavicular joint. Measure the leg distance from the cathode to the xiphoid process with the leg in the anatomical position.

NORMAL VALUES

(Values taken from Daube [2].)

	Mean (msec)	Range (msec)	Distance (cm)	Contralateral Difference (msec)
Ulnar/hypothenar	26.6	21–32	50–76	0–3
Median/thenar	26.4	22–31	57–73	0–3
Tibial/abductor hallucis brevis	48.6	41–57	106–125	0–4
Peroneal/extensor digitorum brevis	47.4	38–57	102–128	0–4

Each lab should develop its own set of normal F-wave latencies which should take both age and limb length into account.

REFERENCES

1. Fisher, Morris A. *Minimonograph #13: Physiology and Clinical Use of the F Response.* Rochester, Minn.: American Association of Electromyography and Electrodiagnosis. June, 1980.
2. Lambert, E. H., and Daube, J. R. (Chairmen). *Special Course #16: Clinical Electromyography.* American Academy of Neurology Meeting, Chicago, Ill., April 23–28, 1979.
3. Mayer, R. F., and Feldman, R. G. Observations on the nature of the F-wave in man. *Neurology* (Minneap.) 17:147, 1967.

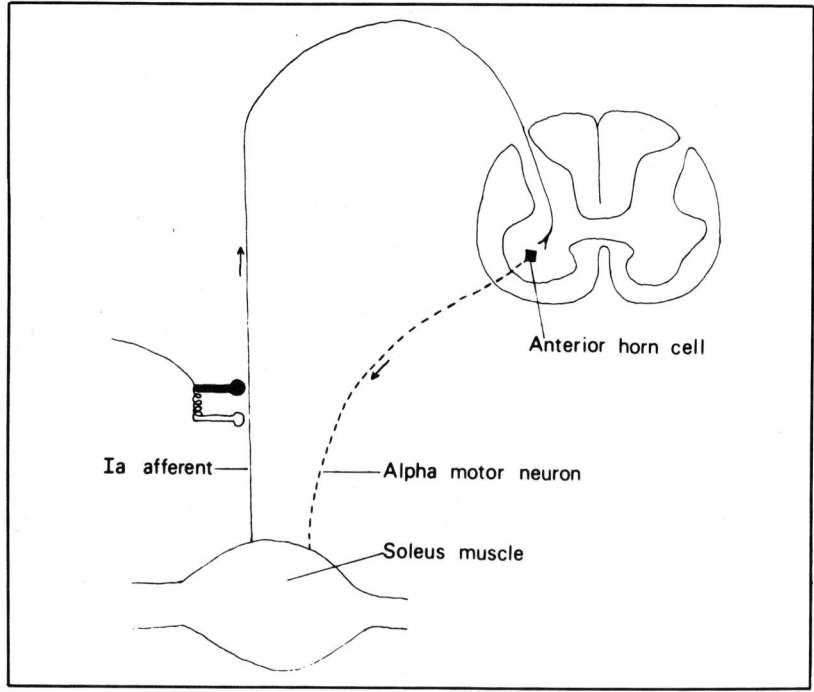

Figure 16-1
*Diagrammatic representation of stimulation of the posterior tibial nerve to elicit the H-reflex. Note that the cathode is **proximal** to the anode.*

Chapter 16 The H-Reflex

ANATOMY AND PHYSIOLOGY

The *H-reflex* is elicited by stimulation of IA afferents in a mixed nerve that evokes a monosynaptic reflex contraction in the same muscle from which these IA (muscle spindle) afferents arise (Fig. 16-1). A minimal stimulus is used to minimize the effect of antidromic stimulation of the motor fibers of the nerve, since antidromic action potentials will obliterate efferent potentials in the same axon or generate an F-wave when a supramaximal stimulus is reached. The threshold for the H-reflex is usually lower than that for the M-response. Starting at low levels of stimulation, the amplitude of the H-reflex should decrease as the intensity of the stimulus is increased after the M-response appears. By the time a supramaximal stimulus intensity for the M-response is reached, the H-reflex should be gone (Fig. 16-2). However, in some persons the H-reflex is seen at the same time as the onset of the M-response. In these cases the amplitude of the H-reflex may increase for a time. The H-reflex will then diminish and will be gone by the time the supramaximal stimulus intensity for the M-response is reached.

In adults the H-reflex is usually recorded in the soleus muscle. It differs from the ankle jerk only in that the IA afferents are stimulated directly rather than by the stretching or vibration of muscle spindles. However, H-reflexes can sometimes be recorded from other muscles in certain situations, and must be distinguished from the F-wave. The latencies of the H-reflex and F-wave tend to be very similar.

APPLICATIONS

The study of the H-reflex provides a way to assess conduction in the

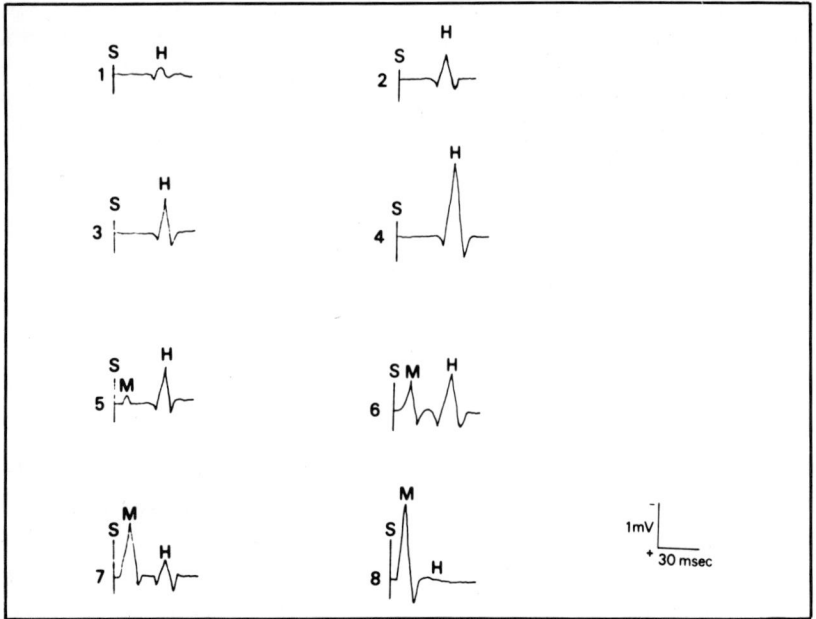

Figure 16-2
Effect of increasing stimulus strength on H-reflex from subthreshold (1) to supramaximal (8). The H-reflex is usually of maximum amplitude just prior to the appearance of the M-response and then disappears with supramaximal stimulation. (S = stimulus, M = M response, H = H-reflex.)

proximal segments of both motor and sensory axons as well as an assessment of the excitability of the anterior horn cell pool.

PROCEDURE

1. Set the gain at 0.5 to 1.0 mV per centimeter with sweep speed at 5 to 10 msec per centimeter.
2. The recording electrode (G_1) is placed over the soleus muscle just medial to the tibia, equidistant between the tibial tubercle and the medial malleolus. The G_2 electrode is placed over the medial aspect of the Achilles tendon just proximal to the superior aspect of the medial malleolus. The ground is between G_1 and G_2 (Fig. 16-3).
3. With the stimulating cathode **proximal** to the anode (Fig. 16-4), stimuli just greater than that required to evoke a minimal M-response are applied to the posterior tibial nerve at the apex of the

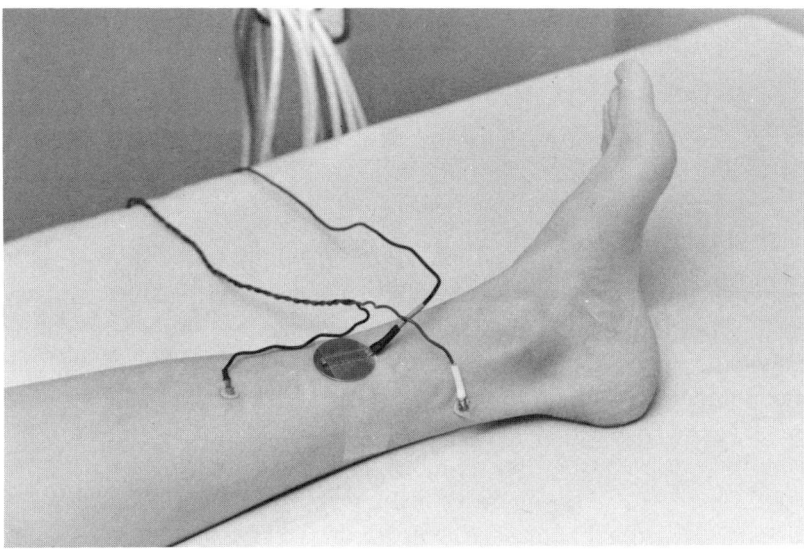

Figure 16-3
Recording electrode placement for the H-reflex.

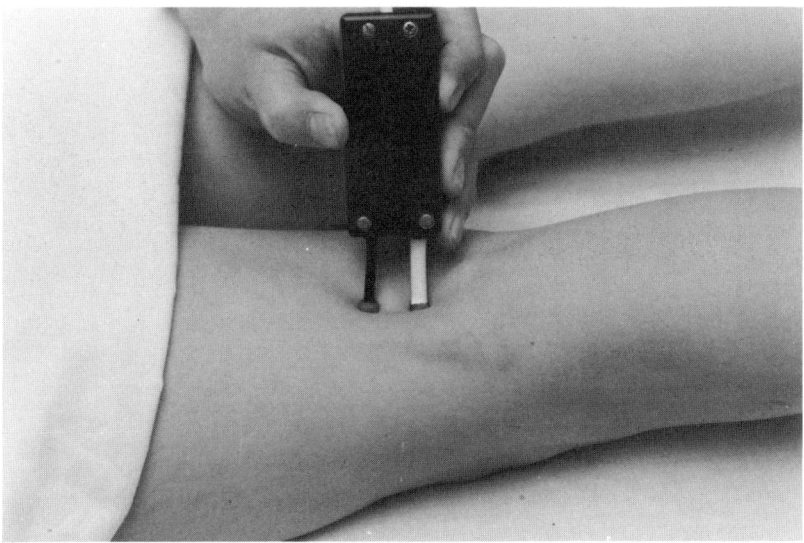

Figure 16-4
Stimulation electrode placement for stimulation of the posterior tibial nerve to elicit the H-reflex. Note that the cathode is **proximal** *to the anode.*

popliteal fossa. The desired frequency to obtain a maximal H-wave amplitude with a minimal M-wave amplitude is every two seconds or less. A series of measurements is made to obtain the shortest reproducible H-wave latency. If the stimulus is increased to near supramaximal, the H-reflex should be reduced or eliminated.

NORMAL VALUES

The normal latency values [1] are distance dependent. The mean latency for the H-reflex is about 29 msec when the distance from the stimulating cathode to the xiphoid process is from 66 to 85 cm and the distance from the stimulating cathode to the G_1 electrode is from 19 to 25 cm. The range of the H-reflex latency for these distances is from 25 to 36 msec. The difference between the H-reflex latencies recorded from each leg should be no more than 3 msec if the amplitude of the reflex and the distances described above are comparable. The parameters of the normal H-reflex are summarized below:

Threshold	Lower than for M-response
Latency	28.9 ± 0.7 msec (decreases with more proximal stimulation)
Amplitude	Largest response 2 to 10 mV
Configuration	Triphasic with a large negative phase

REFERENCE

1. Lambert, E. H., and Daube, J. R. (Chairmen). *Special Course #16: Clinical Electromyography.* American Academy of Neurology Meeting, Chicago, Ill., April 23–28, 1979.

Chapter 17 Slow Repetitive Supramaximal Stimulation of a Motor Nerve

ANATOMY AND PHYSIOLOGY

With repetitive supramaximal stimulation, it is assumed that an increase or decrease in the amplitude of the action potential results from an increase or decrease in the number of muscle fibers responding to successive stimuli, if the cause is a defect in neuromuscular transmission or a failure of conduction in the nerve [2]. In myasthenia gravis the initial evoked muscle action potential (EMAP) is of near-normal amplitude if a maximal or supramaximal stimulus intensity is used. Successive action potentials decrease in amplitude until the fourth through sixth response with a total decrement of at least 10 percent. Three seconds after a thirty-second, strong, voluntary isometric contraction of the muscle, the amplitude of the response is increased and the progressive decline during repetitive stimulation at a slow rate is diminished or absent (postactivation facilitation). About two minutes after the strong contraction, the defect of neuromuscular transmission is more marked than in the well-rested muscle (postactivation exhaustion).

In contrast, the first EMAP in patients with Lambert-Eaton syndrome is consistently of low amplitude even with supramaximal stimulation. At slow stimulation rates (less than 10 per second) there is a decrement of the next four to ten EMAPs. Thirty seconds of isometric exercise produces immediate facilitation (combined with attenuation or loss of the decremental response), but when the test is repeated two minutes after exercise, the amplitude of the EMAP has returned to control values and the decremental response has returned.

The decremental response is strikingly temperature dependent [1]. It is important to maintain the muscle temperature between 35 C and

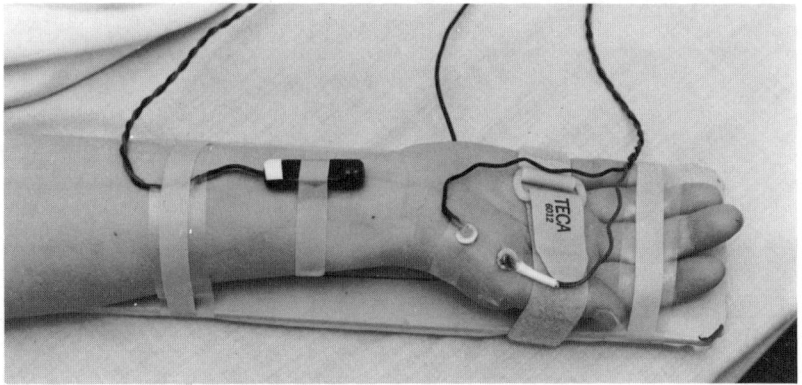

Figure 17-1
Electrode placement for repetitive stimulation of the median nerve. Note that the small bipolar electrode is used for stimulation so that it can also be immobilized.

37°C, because the decremental response to repetitive stimulation and increased decremental response after exercise may disappear if the myasthenic muscle is cooled by only a few degrees. There are many variations possible with different rates of stimulation, exercise, and ischemia. The responses to these circumstances and to prolonged slow stimulation or faster rates of stimulation are beyond the scope of this discussion.

APPLICATIONS

Study of slow repetitive supramaximal stimulation of a motor nerve is useful in the diagnosis of myasthenia gravis and the myasthenic syndrome.

PROCEDURE

1. Apply electrode for median NCV determination (Fig. 4-2).
2. Immobilize the extremity so that contractions of the abductor pollicis brevis are isometric (Fig. 17-1).
3. Stimuli should be supramaximal (at least 25% above maximal).
4. Stimulate 3 times at 2 per second, resting the muscle at least 15 seconds between trains of three stimuli if more than one series of three stimuli is used.
   a. Test the muscle at rest.
   b. Test the muscle 3 seconds after a 30 second voluntary isometric contraction (postactivation facilitation).

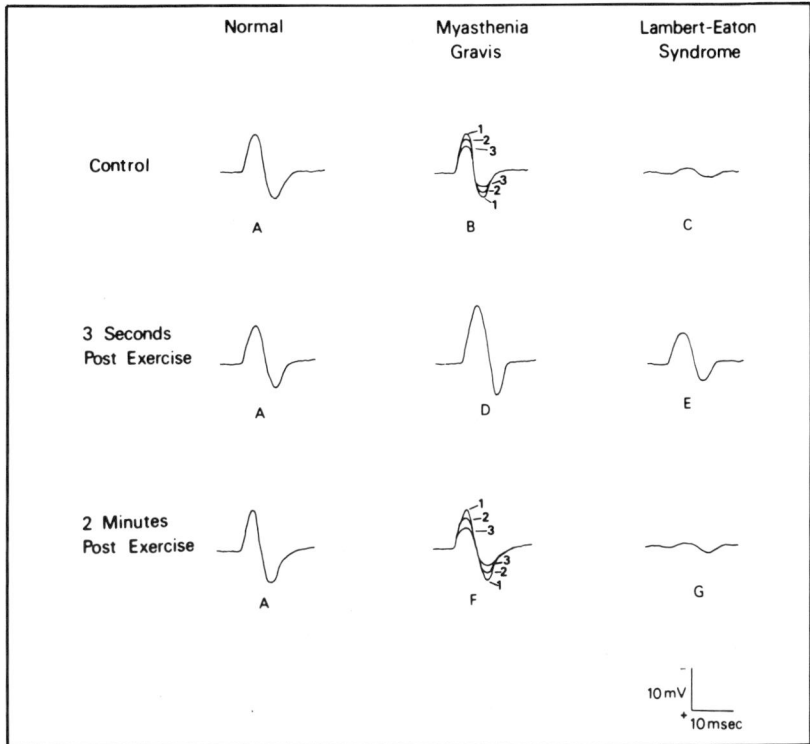

Figure 17-2
Two per second repetitive supramaximal stimulation. A. No change. B. Decrement with repetitive stimulation. C. Initial EMAP smaller than normal; decremental response present but cannot be seen due to low amplification. D. Postexercise increase in amplitude of EMAP combined with loss of decremental response. E. Marked postexercise increase in amplitude of EMAP combined with loss of decremental response. F. Decremental response is now of greater magnitude than control (pre-exercise). G. Return of amplitude of EMAP to control value; again, decremental response is present but cannot be seen at this amplification.

c. Test the muscle 2 minutes after the 30 second voluntary isometric contraction (postactivation exhaustion).

NORMAL VALUES

A reliable response to repetitive stimulation is reproducible and demonstrates a smooth progression of the decremental changes in action potential amplitude (Fig. 17-2). A decrement in amplitude of 8 to 10 percent or greater may be significant [2]. Absence of decrement does not exclude a diagnosis of myasthenia gravis, because only about 65 percent of patients with myasthenia gravis show a decrement in the hand muscles at slow rates of stimulation. The normal amplitude of the negative component of the EMAP from the abductor pollicis is approximately 10 mV with a range of 5 to 20 mV.

REFERENCES

1. Borenstein, S., and Desmedt, J. E. New Diagnostic Procedures in Myasthenia Gravis. In J. E. Desmedt (Ed.), *New Developments in EMG and Clinical Neurophysiology*. Volume 1. Basel: Karger, 1973.
2. Goodgold, J., and Eberstein, A. *Electrodiagnosis of Neuromuscular Diseases* (2nd ed.). Baltimore: Williams & Wilkins, 1977.

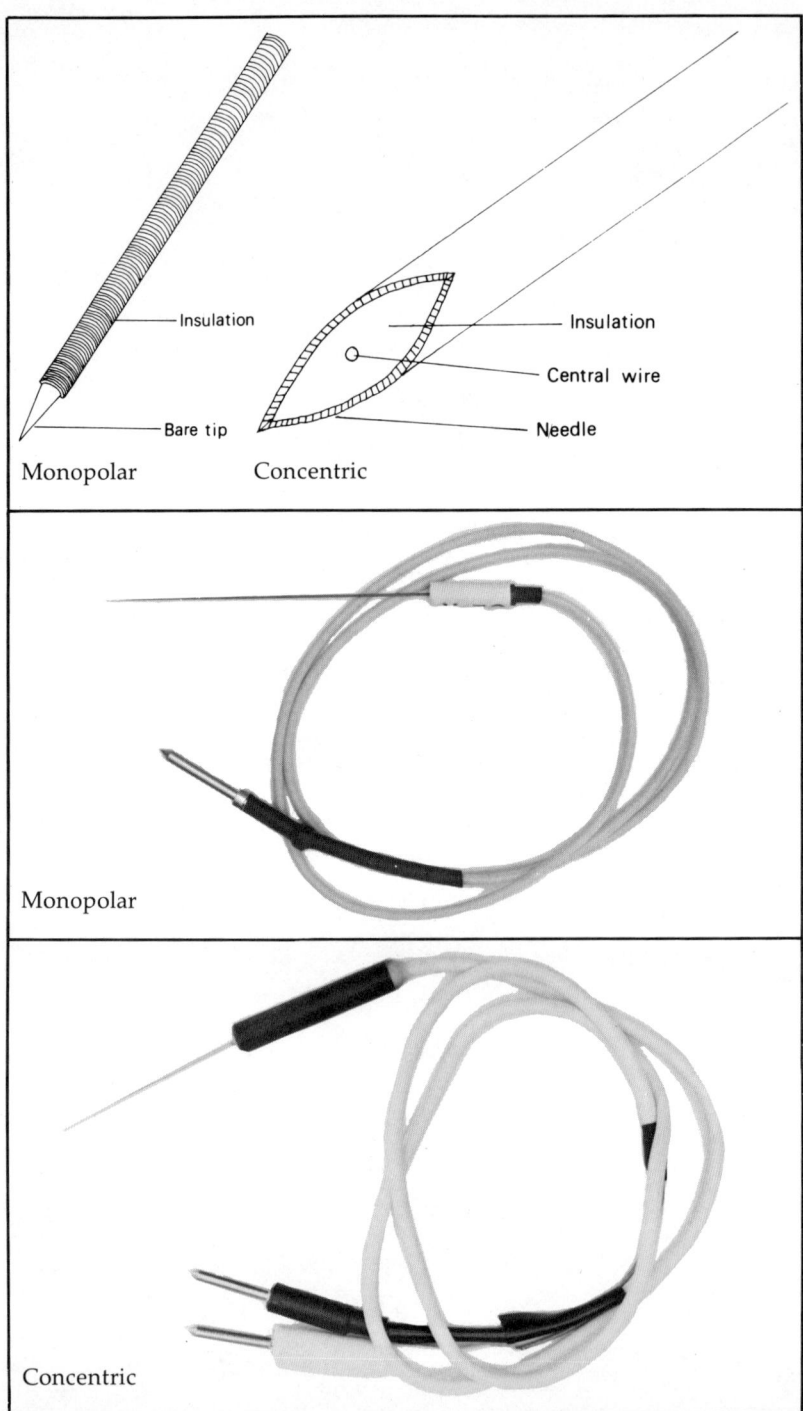

Figure 18-1
Monopolar and concentric electrodes.

Chapter 18 The EMG Examination

Because there are over 430 skeletal muscles in the human body and patchy involvement of muscle may exist in some neuromuscular diseases, it is impossible to standardize completely the "needle" examination. The discussion that follows attempts to highlight the major aspects of clinical EMG, since it is understood that the needle examination is really learned only by working with an accomplished electromyographer.

Two main types of needle electrodes (Fig. 18-1) are used in electromyographic recording: the *concentric* (coaxial) and the *monopolar*. Concentric electrodes consist of an outer cannula or needle through which a single insulated wire with a bare tip passes. The outer needle may also be insulated, except at its tip. The inner wire serves as the recording electrode and the outer cannula as the reference electrode. A separate ground is used. Monopolar needle electrodes are simply solid electrodes (needles) covered with some type of insulation (usually Teflon) except at the tip. This electrode serves as the recording electrode; a second reference electrode (either needle or surface) must be placed nearby. A separate ground is also used.

The duration of the major spike potential (see below under Exertional Activity) is longer with the monopolar electrode; however, the total duration of the motor unit action potential (MUAP) is very nearly the same as that recorded with either type of electrode [9]. Also, amplitude tends to be somewhat higher when it is recorded by the concentric electrode. The major problem with the concentric electrode, however, is that it causes the patient more pain than the monopolar electrode. Therefore, although one tends to record somewhat sharper motor units with the concentric electrodes, many investigators prefer the Teflon-

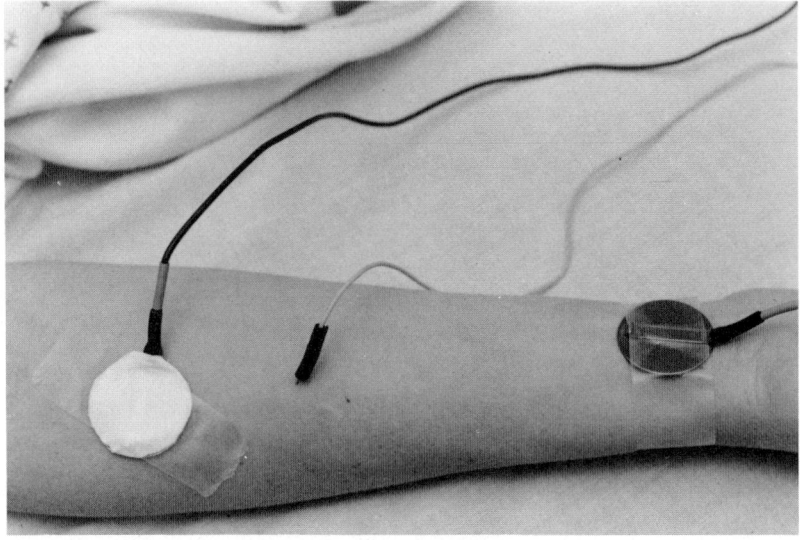

Figure 18-2
Electrode placement for the EMG examination of the muscles of the forearm. The monopolar electrode is in the brachioradialis.

coated monopolar electrode because almost every muscle in the body can be studied with little discomfort to the patient.

In most routine EMG examinations a monopolar needle electrode can be used as the recording electrode (G_1). A flat surface disc electrode is used for the reference electrode (G_2) and another disc electrode for the ground. The ground electrode is usually placed over a bony prominence and the reference electrode (G_2) is placed near the muscle to be tested (Fig. 18-2). Placement of the ground or reference, or both, may have to be changed during an examination to help minimize baseline artifact. There are no stimulation electrodes.

Three basic measurements of the myoneural relationship are routinely explored during a needle examination: *insertional activity, spontaneous activity,* and *exertional activity,* which is activity evoked by voluntary muscular effort made by the patient.

INSERTIONAL ACTIVITY

As the needle electrode enters or is moved within a muscle, fibers are mechanically stimulated, cut, and injured. These alterations of the mus-

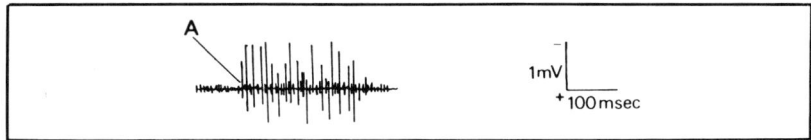

Figure 18-3
Normal insertional activity (A = point of needle insertion or cessation of needle movement).

cle cells give rise to bursts of potentials. A single burst should not last more than 300 msec after the movement of the needle ceases (Fig. 18-3). Potentials occurring after this period (300 msec) are a type of spontaneous activity and are usually abnormal. *Prolonged* insertional activity is abnormal insertional activity.

SPONTANEOUS ACTIVITY

Spontaneous activity occurs after insertional activity has ceased, although the two may merge in a muscle that displays spontaneous activity. Spontaneous activity is usually abnormal, but there are some exceptions.

Abnormal Spontaneous Activity

Fibrillations

Fibrillation potentials (Fig. 18-4) recorded outside the zone of innervation (see below under Normal Spontaneous Activity) have an initial phase that is positive and a total of two or three phases. The interpotential interval should be regular with a firing rate of one to ten per second. Fibrillation potentials originate from a single muscle fiber.

Fibrillations are recorded when the needle is outside the muscle fiber and are sometimes referred to as extracellularly recorded injury potentials. These injury potentials are the result of muscle cell membrane irritability and are seen most often in denervated muscle (e.g., neuropathy) but may also be seen in myopathies of multiple etiologies (e.g., progressive muscular dystrophy, polymyositis, hyperkalemic familial periodic paralysis) [2]. In rare instances fibrillation potentials are also recorded in normal muscles; their isolated appearance is *not* pathognomonic of neuropathy or myopathy.

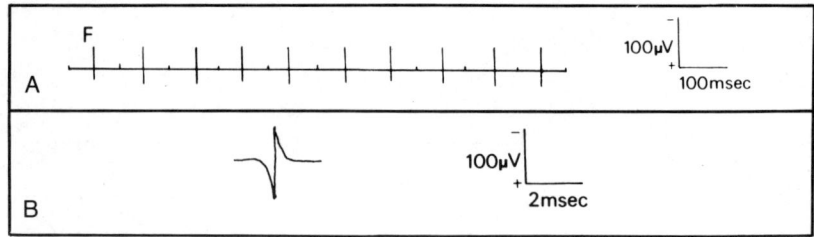

Figure 18-4
(A) *fibrillations* (F) *at an average rate of ten per second and a single fibrillation potential* (B).

Potentials having some of the characteristics of fibrillations are occasionally seen; they have irregular interpotential intervals. These irregularly firing potentials are probably best disregarded, for they are often artifacts of the technique rather than true indicators of muscle cell membrane irritability. Some examples are discussed below under Normal Spontaneous Activity.

The essential characteristics of fibrillation potentials are as follows:

Amplitude	20–300 μV
Duration	1–5 msec (average 2.7 msec)
Frequency	1–10 per second (occasionally up to 30 per second)
Firing Interval	Regular
Sound	"rain on the roof" or "high-pitched clicks"
Configuration	Diphasic or triphasic with initial deflection positive (downward)

Positive sharp waves

Positive sharp waves may be considered as intracellularly recorded injury potentials that are recorded when the needle electrode is within or very near the muscle fiber (cell) that is discharging [2]. They are usually seen accompanying fibrillation potentials. They are diphasic potentials with an abrupt initial positive deflection followed by a slow negative decay (Fig. 18-5). On occasion, movement of the EMG needle will demonstrate a transition from fibrillations to positive waves in a single fiber. The characteristics of positive sharp waves are summarized below:

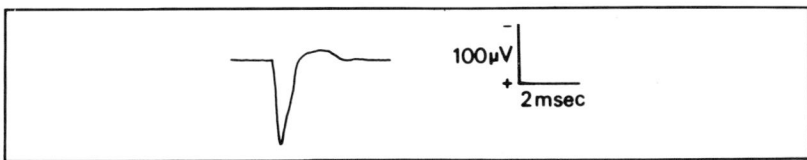

Figure 18-5
A positive sharp wave.

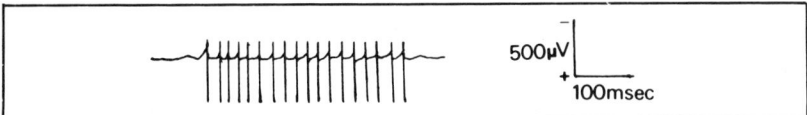

Figure 18-6
Complex repetitive discharges.

Amplitude (usual)	120 μV ± 45 μV
Amplitude (extreme)	Up to 3 mV (rarely)
Duration	Usually greater than 10 msec (up to 100 msec due to prolonged negative phase)
Frequency	Usually 10 per second (range 2–100)
Firing Interval	Variable; usually regular
Configuration	Diphasic; initial abrupt positive deflection followed by gradual return to baseline (large first phase) with minimal overshoot (small second phase)
Sound	Dull, popping

Positive sharp waves may be present only in the first few seconds after the needle is inserted or movement ceases. They are most commonly seen in denervated muscle but can be observed in myopathies as well. They are *not* seen in normal muscle, but they otherwise have the same implications as fibrillations. Care must be taken to have the muscle completely relaxed, because motor units at a distance from the needle electrode may superficially resemble positive sharp waves.

Complex repetitive discharges

These extended trains of potentials are characterized by their frequency, which is rapid (20–150 per second) [12]. The amplitude, duration, and form (usually polyphasic) of the potentials are variable but identical within any single train (Fig. 18-6). They may be seen in neuropathies and myopathies. Onset and termination are abrupt.

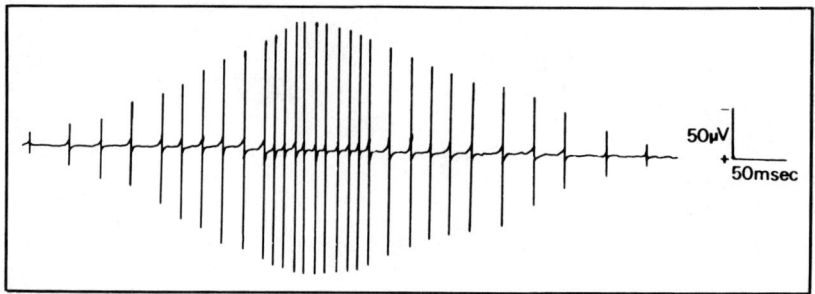
Figure 18-7
Idealized myotonic discharge.

Electrical myotonia

Electrical myotonia is a special type of high-frequency discharge and is seen in myotonic dystrophy, myotonia congenita, and paramyotonia congenita [12]. True electrical myotonia is characterized by high-frequency discharges that vary in frequency and amplitude. This waxing and waning (up to 150 per second and down to 20 per second) of the discharge frequency, coupled with a parallel variation in amplitude, gives a characteristic "dive-bomber" sound over the loudspeaker. After the cessation of a voluntary contraction, these waxing and waning potentials may persist for several minutes (Fig. 18-7).

Fasciculations

A fasciculation (Fig. 18-8) is the nonvolitional contraction of a group of muscle fibers that may cause both visible movements of the skin and movement of a small joint. Fasciculations are most commonly seen in patients with proximal neuropathies (e.g., motor neuron disease, irritation of spinal nerve roots) but may occur in those with thyrotoxicosis and also in normal individuals, especially in the calf muscles and the small muscles of the hands and feet. A summary of the characteristics of fasciculations is given below:

Duration	3–16 msec
Amplitude	300 μV–5 mV
Configuration	Diphasic to polyphasic
Repetition Frequency	1–50 per *minute*

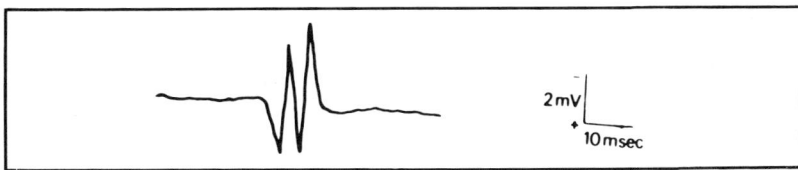

Figure 18-8
A fasciculation.

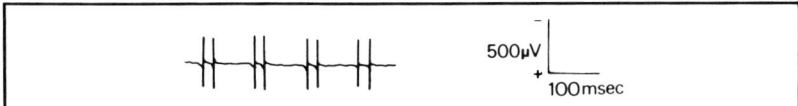

Figure 18-9
Grouped motor unit discharges.

Firing Interval   Irregular
Sound   Dull pop

Fasciculations resemble single motor unit potentials in appearance. "Benign" fasciculations tend to be more frequent (averaging about 1 per second), whereas "malignant" fasciculations tend to be less frequent (averaging about 1 every *three* seconds). However, in a given individual it may be difficult to distinguish between fasciculations and single motor unit potentials without corroborative positive or negative information [2].

Myokymia

Myokymia is a spontaneous slow contraction of small bands of muscle fibers that gives a rippling appearance to the overlying skin [12]. Myokymia represents a sustained contraction which should be distinguished from the single twitch of a fasciculation. Myokymia is rare, but has been reported in cases of thyrotoxicosis, cramp, hyperhidrosis, myotonia-like contractions, muscular atrophy, tetany, uremia, and nerve compression; it also appears in some normal persons. Facial myokymia has also been seen in patients with multiple sclerosis and pontine gliomas. Electrically, myokymia consists of repetitive, grouped bursts of 2 to 200 identical motor unit potentials occurring at a rate of about 50 per second (Fig. 18-9). They are sometimes referred to as *grouped* or *iterative motor unit discharges*.

Cramp

A cramp is a transient, involuntary, painful muscular contraction which may result from unaccustomed exertion, sodium depletion, uremia, hypocalcemia, alkalosis, or drugs, but whose origin is most often unexplained. The EMG reflects the full interference pattern of maximal effort or may demonstrate only a few rapidly firing motor units in the vicinity of the needle.

Contracture

A contracture must be differentiated from a cramp. An electrically silent shortening of muscles induced by exertion, contractures are seen in McArdle's disease, phosphofructokinase deficiency, or other glycogen storage diseases of muscle, and in chronic alcoholism associated with hypokalemia after bouts of heavy drinking [12]. The muscle is shortened, tense, tender, and painful, but the contracture is electrically silent. EMG may, therefore, be necessary to distinguish a contracture from a cramp. Clinically, a contracture lasts from a few minutes to several hours; severe, brief episodes of muscle pain are usually electrically active cramps.

The stiff-man syndrome

The stiff-man syndrome is a strange and rare disorder in which a symmetrical continuous stiffness of the muscles develops, leaving the patient rigid in extension [12]. The EMG reveals continuous, normal-appearing motor unit activity that persists in the absence of effort, but disappears with sleep. These persistent tonic contractions represent hyperactivity of the gamma system and can be relieved by diazepam.

Neuromyotonia

Neuromyotonia or the "continuous muscle fiber activity" syndrome causes muscle stiffness and difficulty with voluntary movement [12]. The EMG at rest reveals dysrhythmic discharges which are a mixture of motor unit activity and low-amplitude short-duration potentials with intervening silent periods of 10 to 20 sec. Neuromyotonia persists during general anesthesia or after nerve block. Motor and sensory nerve conductions tend to be at the lower limits of normal with prolonged

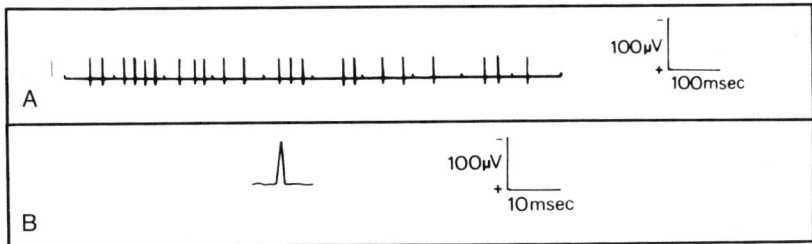

Figure 18-10
A. Miniature end-plate potentials. B. A single MEPP.

distal latencies. This condition is improved by the administration of phenytoin or carbamazepine.

Normal Spontaneous Activity

Normal muscle at rest is electrically silent except in the zone of innervation of the muscle where at least two types of end-plate noise may be identified [2].

Miniature end-plate potentials

These high-frequency spontaneous potentials are probably the same as miniature end-plate potentials (MEPP). MEPP are nonpropagated, subthreshold depolarizations (Fig. 18-10). The essential characteristics of MEPP are summarized as follows:

Amplitude	10–100 μV
Duration	1–2 msec
Frequency	10–25 per second
Firing Interval	Irregular
Sound	Seashell held to the ear
Configuration	Diphasic with initial deflection negative

"Nerve" potentials

"Nerve" potentials may represent MEPPs that have been sufficiently augmented to evoke a propagated action potential along a muscle fiber (Fig. 18-11). These potentials are generally associated with the complaint

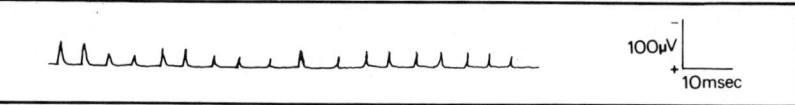

Figure 18-11
"Nerve" potentials.

of pain by the patient and have the following characteristics:

Amplitude	Up to 200 μV
Duration	3–5 msec
Frequency	Up to 50 per second
Firing Interval	Irregular
Sound	Buzzing, crackling
Configuration	Diphasic with initial deflection negative

Both MEPPs and "nerve" potentials disappear with slight movement of the needle. Confusion arises because within the zone of innervation (end-plate zone), fibrillation potentials also have an initial *negative* deflection and are of amplitude and duration similar to those produced by end-plate noise. Therefore, low-amplitude, short-duration potentials within the zone of innervation may be either end-plate noise or fibrillations. Evaluation for fibrillation potentials should be done *outside* of the zone of innervation. The initial deflection of a fibrillation outside of the zone of innervation will be *positive* and end-plate noise should not exist. The zone of innervation is in the region of the motor point of a muscle. Refer to Appendix IX for the locations of motor points of selected muscles [5].

EXERTIONAL ACTIVITY

The single MUAP originates from one motor unit, although it is still uncertain whether the major spike potential of the single motor unit reflects the activity of one or several muscle fibers [2]. A normal MUAP will have an initial positive deflection followed by a very short positive to negative deflection. The duration of this major spike (i.e., the rapid positive to negative deflection) is in the range of 100 to 200 microseconds. With careful electrode placement and a cooperative patient who is able to control a minimal effort, a single MUAP can be displayed on the oscilloscope (Fig. 18-12). It is useful to "freeze" this unit using a delay line and storage for more careful study or photography, or both,

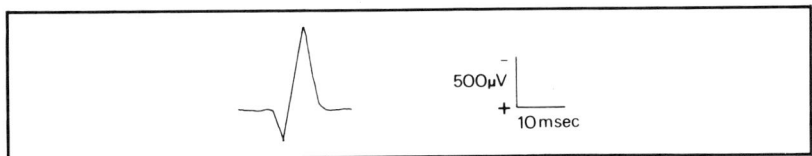

Figure 18-12
A single MUAP.

when first learning to appreciate the enormous range of normal variations of the MUAP. The essential characteristics of the MUAP (Fig. 18-13) are as follows:

Amplitude	300 μV to 5 mV
Duration	3–10 msec; up to 16 msec can be normal
Frequency	Depends on degree of effort and nature of the recruitment (5–50 per second)
Configuration	Usually 2–3 phases; more than 4 is considered polyphasia
Firing Interval	Regular
Sound	Sharp and crisp when the MUAP being studied is generated by fibers very near the tip of the needle electrode

It is necessary to position the EMG needle tip as near as possible to the fiber or fibers generating the major spike potential of the motor unit being studied. As the appropriate fiber is approached, the MUAP will be both seen and heard to sharpen. The amplitude of the major spike will increase, its duration will decrease, and the duration and configuration of the entire MUAP will "normalize." Stated another way, normal MUAPs recorded from a distance may appear abnormal. For example, they may superficially resemble positive waves.

The amplitude, duration, and number of phases of normal MUAPs vary greatly from muscle to muscle. The range of values also varies with electrode type and other circumstances of recording. Amplitude is the most variable MUAP characteristic. Wide ranges of normal amplitude values are observed, and only extremes can be considered abnormal. Amplitude is lower in the extraocular, facial, intercostal, and paraspinous muscles while it is higher in the muscles of the extremities. Duration of the MUAP [1] depends upon the innervation ratio of the nerve

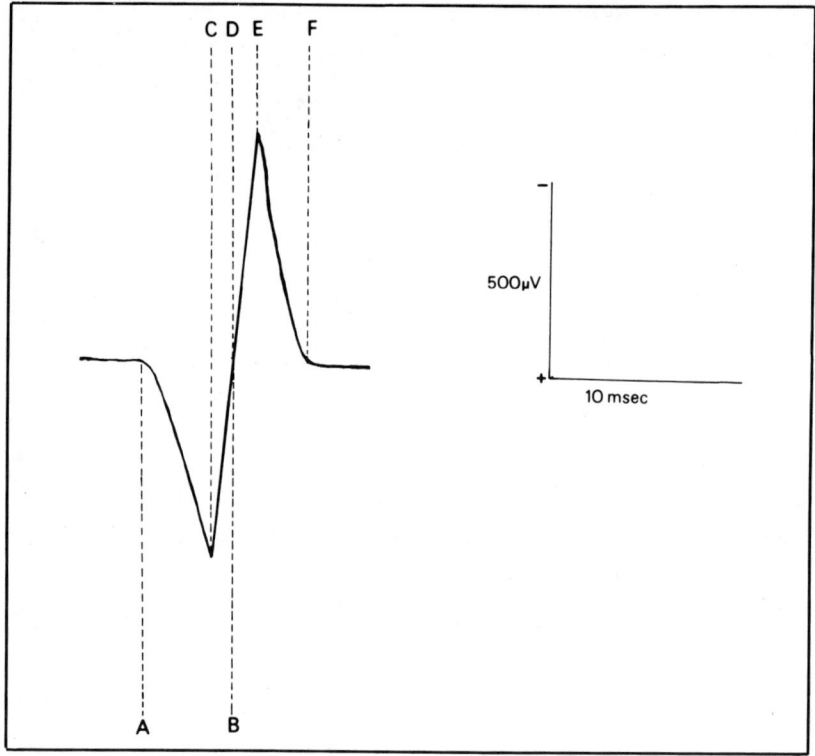

Figure 18-13
Characteristics of a single MUAP (A→B: positive phase; D→F: negative phase; C→E: major spike (amplitude vertical, duration horizontal); A→F: MUAP duration).

and muscle fibers. It is shorter in the facial muscles and longer in the muscles of the extremities (Tables 18-1 and 18-2). The duration of the MUAPs of the facial muscles ranges from about 4.2 msec at birth to approximately 7.4 msec at age 75.

Some degree of polyphasia is a normal phenomenon. It can be detected in about 10 percent of the units of limb muscles such as the deltoid. However, very polyphasic units (up to 12 phases) may be definitely abnormal even if just a few are seen. If the degree of polyphasia observed is mild, 20 to 40 single motor unit potentials must be examined in a single muscle to determine the overall percentage of polyphasic units in a given muscle. Refer to Table 18-3 for a tabulation of degrees of polyphasia for specific muscles [1]. Total mean duration of the MUAP tends to increase with age [1,11]. The percentage of polyphasic units

Table 18-1
Mean Durations of Motor Unit Action Potentials in Upper Extremity Muscles

Age (years)	Deltoid (msec)	Biceps Brachii (msec)	Triceps Brachii (msec)	Opponens Pollicis (msec)	Abductor Digiti Quinti (msec)
0–4	7.9–10.1	6.4–8.2	7.2–9.3	7.1–9.1	8.3–10.6
5–9	8.0–10.8	6.5–8.8	7.3–9.9	7.2–9.8	8.4–11.4
10–14	8.1–11.2	6.6–9.1	7.5–10.3	7.3–10.1	8.5–11.7
15–19	8.6–12.2	7.0–9.9	7.9–11.2	7.8–11.0	9.0–12.8
20–29	9.5–13.2	7.7–10.7	8.7–12.1	8.5–11.9	9.9–13.8
30–39	11.1–14.9	9.0–12.1	10.2–13.7	10.0–13.4	11.6–15.6
40–49	11.8–15.7	9.6–12.8	10.9–14.5	10.7–14.2	12.4–16.5
50–59	12.8–16.7	10.4–13.6	11.8–15.4	11.5–15.1	13.4–17.5
60–69	13.3–17.3	10.8–14.1	12.2–15.9	12.0–15.7	13.9–18.2
70–79	13.7–17.7	11.1–14.4	12.5–16.3	12.3–16.0	14.3–18.6

Source: From F. Buchthal and P. Rosenfalck. Action potential parameters in different human muscles. *Acta Psychiatr. Neurol. Scand.* 30:125, 1955. Used by permission.

Table 18-2
Mean Durations of Motor Unit Action Potentials in Lower Extremity Muscles

Age (years)	Biceps Femoris: Quadriceps (msec)	Gastrocnemius (msec)	Tibialis Anterior (msec)	Peroneus Longus (msec)	Extensor Digitorum Brevis (msec)
0–4	7.2–9.2	6.4–8.2	8.0–10.2	5.8–7.4	6.3–8.1
5–9	7.3–9.9	6.5–8.8	8.1–11.0	5.9–7.9	6.4–8.7
10–14	7.4–10.2	6.6–9.1	8.2–11.3	5.9–8.2	6.5–9.0
15–19	7.8–11.1	7.0–9.9	8.7–12.3	6.3–8.9	6.9–9.8
20–29	8.6–12.0	7.7–10.7	9.6–13.3	6.9–9.6	7.6–10.6
30–39	10.1–13.5	9.0–12.1	11.2–15.1	8.1–10.9	8.9–12.0
40–49	10.7–14.3	9.6–12.8	11.9–15.9	8.6–11.5	9.5–12.7
50–59	11.6–15.2	10.4–13.6	12.9–16.9	9.4–12.2	10.3–13.5
60–69	12.1–15.8	10.8–14.1	13.4–17.5	9.7–12.7	10.7–14.0
70–79	12.4–16.1	11.1–14.4	13.8–17.9	10.0–13.0	11.0–14.3

Source: From F. Buchthal and P. Rosenfalck. Action potential parameters in different human muscles. *Acta Psychiatr. Neurol. Scand.* 30:125, 1955. Used by permission.

Table 18-3
Polyphasic Potentials in Normal Human Muscles

Muscle	Polyphasic Potentials (%)
Biceps brachii	3.5
Biceps femoris	4.5
Gastrocnemius	0.5
Tibialis anterior	8.5
Facial muscles	5.5
Extensor digitorum brevis	12.0

Source: Adapted from F. Buchthal and P. Rosenfalck. Action potential parameters in different human muscles. *Acta Psychiatr. Neurol. Scand.* 30:125, 1955. Used by permission.

also becomes higher as age increases. Age-related amplitude changes are more variable. Table 18-4 summarizes these changes in the abductor digiti quinti of the hand and the biceps brachii.

The "average" motor unit will begin firing at a rate of about 5 per second (200-msec inter-MUAP onset interval). The interpotential interval is regular with a smooth, continuous effort. This interval with minimum effort is best appreciated with a sweep speed of 100 msec per centimeter (Fig. 18-14).

This rate of firing will increase up to 25 to 50 per second (20–40 msec interpotential interval) with increased effort (Fig. 18-15).

In normal muscle when a single MUAP reaches a firing rate of about 10 to 15 per second (66–100 msec interpotential interval), an additional motor unit is "recruited" to help create the additional force of contraction required to increase effort (Fig. 18-16). The rate of firing at which recruitment occurs varies from muscle to muscle and is called the *recruitment interval* [7]. Onset and recruitment intervals are discussed in more detail below in conjunction with the interference pattern.

At a sweep speed of 10 msec per centimeter, a single motor unit potential pattern is normally recorded when a patient exerts a minimal effort. One or two MUAPs are clearly seen to be firing at rates of from 4 to 20 times per second. With maximal effort, many motor units are activated (recruited) to fire at rates of 25 to 50 times per second and single MUAPs cannot be visually identified because of extensive overlapping. A complete interference pattern occurs and obliterates the baseline. Recruitment is said to be normal when a complete interference

Table 18-4
Variation of Duration, Amplitude, and Configuration of the MUAP (Concentric Electrode)

Age	Mean Duration ± Standard Error of the Mean (msec)	Mean Voltage (μV)	Polyphasic Potentials in > 4 phases (%)
Abductor Digiti Quinti			
3 months	5.8 ± 0.1	78 ± 12	0.6
16–23 years	9.4 ± 0.25	360 ± 20	3.3
26–40 years	9.1 ± 0.25	....	2.0
47–52 years	9.0 ± 0.3	....	4.7
61–80 years	10.1 ± 0.35	330 ± 50	4.4
Biceps Brachii			
3 months	7.7 ± 0.3	96 ± 7	6.0
16–23 years	10.3 ± 0.2	175 ± 20	2.8
26–40 years	10.9 ± 0.45	....	4.9
47–52 years	11.3 ± 0.35	....	4.9
61–80 years	12.7 ± 0.25	290 ± 40	3.8

Source: Adapted from G. Sacco, F. Buchthal, and P. Rosenfalck. Motor unit potentials at different ages. *Arch. Neurol.* 6:44, 1962. Copyright 1962, American Medical Association.

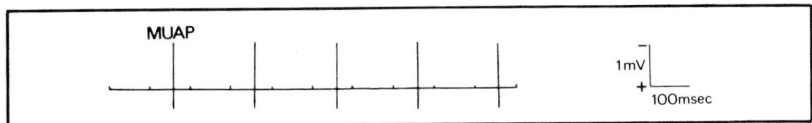

Figure 18-14
MUAP onset interval of 200 msec.

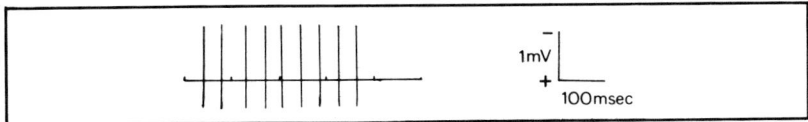

Figure 18-15
The motor unit increases its rate of firing with increased effort.

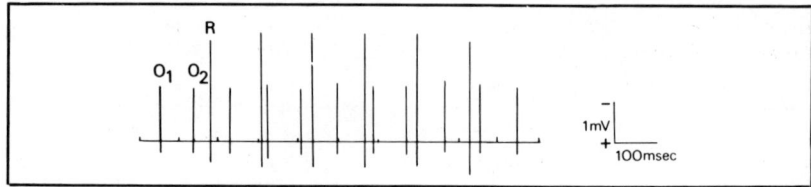

Figure 18-16
Recruitment interval. (O = *original motor unit*, R = *recruited motor unit*, O_1 to O_2 = *recruitment interval.*)

pattern occurs. There are various degrees of partial or incomplete interference patterns between these two extremes (Fig. 18-17).

Because of scattered single fiber loss with *relative* preservation of the motor units in myopathic states, many motor units must fire to generate minimal power; therefore, a complete interference pattern is often seen with minimal effort. It is relatively easy to recognize the complete interference pattern of myopathy with its brief small abundant polyphasic potentials (BSAPPs) generated by minimal to modest effort (Fig. 18-18). Recruitment is said to be increased.

Analysis of the incomplete interference pattern is much more difficult. Loss of motor units, as in a neuropathy, will cause an incomplete interference pattern (decreased recruitment) with what seems to be maximal effort, but effort may be compromised by pain, fear, misunderstanding, hysteria, malingering, or upper motor neuron disease. Also, interference patterns tend to be incomplete in the larger leg muscles, especially the gastrocnemius and soleus muscles. Effort cannot be assumed to be full unless the rate of firing of the MUAPs is clearly rapid (30–50 times per second). The rate of firing of individual units can be difficult to determine when several are firing at once. Long experience attending to rates of firing can make a determination possible, but it is probably prudent *not* to accept an incomplete interference pattern as diagnostic of motor unit loss unless other evidence is forthcoming. If several distinct motor units can definitely be seen to be firing at 30 to 50 per second, there is probably some decrease in the total number of motor units, but decreased recruitment alone is *not* pathognomonic of neuropathy.

If instructed to give attention to auditory and visual cues, a patient usually can learn quickly to activate a single MUAP and maintain its firing. Analysis of the interspike interval of a single MUAP at a minimal

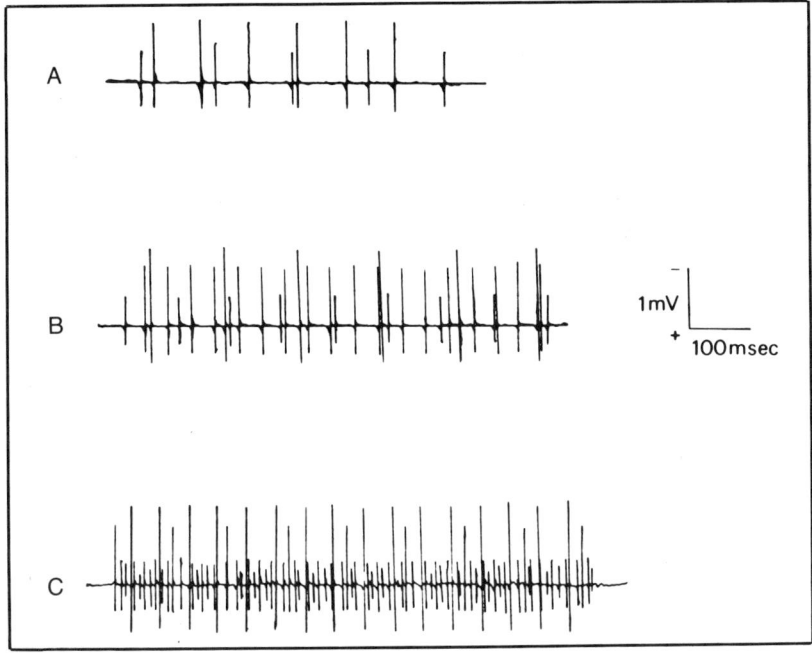

Figure 18-17
Normal interference patterns. A. Single motor unit interference pattern (minimal effort). B. Incomplete interference pattern (modest effort). C. Complete interference pattern (maximal effort).

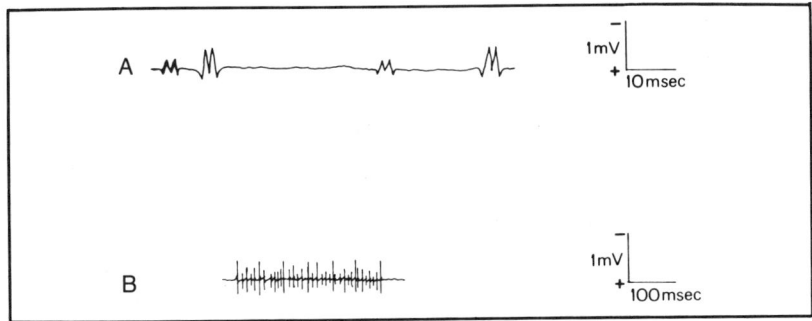

Figure 18-18
Myopathy: two MUAPs activated with least possible effort (A) and complete interference pattern with less than maximal effort (B).

level of effort is useful in distinguishing the normal state from myopathies and neuropathies. Moreover, with a gradual increase in effort a second MUAP will be recruited when the rate of firing of the initial MUAP reaches a certain frequency and the interspike interval has therefore shortened to a certain degree. The interspike interval at the onset of firing is known as the *onset interval* (Fig. 18-14), and the interspike interval of the *initial* MUAP at the time of recruitment of a second motor unit is known as the *recruitment interval* (Fig. 18-16). Onset and recruitment intervals vary from muscle to muscle and individual to individual (Table 18-5). The average normal onset interval is 132 msec (MUAP firing at 7½ times per second) and the average normal recruitment interval is 90 msec (original MUAP firing at 11 times per second).

In both myopathies and neuropathies the onset and recruitment intervals tend to be shorter [8]. In both of these pathological conditions the motor unit starts firing at a faster rate, and there is an even faster firing rate (compared to normal) at the time of recruitment of a second motor unit (Table 18-6). Analysis of onset and recruitment intervals is especially useful when one is faced with an incomplete interference pattern which is difficult to interpret in isolation.

Attention to onset intervals and recruitment intervals is also good practice in training the ear to appreciate different firing rates of MUAPs. The sweep speed is usually set at 100 msec per centimeter for this determination. If the interference pattern is complete only with maximal effort and onset and recruitment intervals are normal, significant neuropathy or myopathy is unlikely (Table 18-7). Moreover, weakness from hysteria, malingering, or pain is characterized by normal single motor unit activity at minimal effort. The careful analysis of motor unit control with minimal effort is often helpful in sorting out the type of weakness present. Obviously, these results must be interpreted in the light of other EMG and NCV findings in the individual patient.

The EMG analysis of upper motor neuron lesions is more complex. Positive waves and fibrillation potentials are reported in patients with spinal cord injuries from various causes and hemiplegia due to vascular disease [4]. These findings occur in the muscles innervated by spinal segments below the level of the spinal cord lesion and do not follow a segmental or peripheral nerve distribution. These signs of muscle cell membrane hyperirritability may begin to appear about 15 days after the spinal cord is injured and are generally no longer present after 12 months have passed.

Table 18-5
Onset and Recruitment Intervals in Normal Human Muscle

Muscle	Onset Intervals (mean ± SD in msec)	Recruitment Intervals (mean ± SD in msec)
All facial muscles	86 ± 29	40 ± 16
Deltoid	116 ± 23	84 ± 16
Biceps	124 ± 21	86 ± 14
Triceps	132 ± 36	84 ± 17
Brachioradialis	116 ± 22	78 ± 18
Pronator teres	132 ± 38	88 ± 19
First dorsal interosseous	142 ± 39	98 ± 21
Vastus lateralis	126 ± 30	88 ± 18
Gluteus maximus	128 ± 30	88 ± 16
Tibialis anterior	124 ± 26	90 ± 13
Biceps femoris	132 ± 29	92 ± 16
Medial gastrocnemius	156 ± 29	110 ± 23
Extensor digitorum brevis	138 ± 29	98 ± 13
All muscles	132 ± 32	90 ± 19

Source: Adapted from J. H. Petajan and B. A. Philip. Frequency control of motor unit action potentials. *Electroencephalogr. Clin. Neurophysiol.* 27:66, 1969. Used by permission.

Table 18-6
Onset and Recruitment Intervals in Neuropathy and Myopathy

	Mean (± SD in msec)	Range (msec)
Neuropathy	OI 48 ± 17	15–110
	RI 36 ± 12	10–65
Myopathy	OI 65 ± 11	40–112
	RI 45 ± 8	20–58
Normal	OI 132 ± 32	76–236
	RI 90 ± 19	44–164

OI = onset interval; RI = recruitment interval
Source: Adapted from J. H. Petajan. Clinical electromyographic studies of diseases of the motor unit. *Electroencephalogr. Clin. Neurophysiol.* 36:395, 1974. Used by permission.

Table 18-7
Exertional Activity of Motor Units

	Interference Pattern	Onset Interval (msec)	Recruitment Interval (msec)
Normal	Complete with maximal effort	132	90
Neuropathy	Incomplete with maximal effort	48	36
Myopathy	Complete with minimal to modest effort	65	45

In the patient with hemiplegia secondary to a vascular stroke, fibrillations and positive waves begin to appear about one week after the ictus; they may persist in the small muscles of the hands and feet for more than a year. These injury potentials are more commonly found in the upper extremity than in the lower extremity and in both regions are more common distally than proximally. This pattern of distribution parallels the typical pattern of greatest weakness in a cerebral infarction with middle cerebral artery distribution. Positive waves and fibrillation potentials apparently occur without coexistent lower motor neuron injury.

Spontaneous firing of motor units in the antigravity muscles often takes place. The rate of motor unit firing can be increased by passively stretching the muscles; with passive shortening of the muscle, the rate will decrease. This "spontaneous" activity reflects the nonvolitional increase in tone caused by many upper motor neuron lesions that makes complete relaxation impossible.

The nature of residual voluntary activity in upper motor neuron disease is also interesting. This activity is characterized by a long latency from onset of effort to onset of recordable motor unit activity. A high level of subjective effort often seems to accompany this latent period. When the motor units do begin to fire, they fire at a more rapid rate than normal; therefore, the onset interval is shorter than normal. Although an almost complete interference pattern may be generated, this burst of activity is brief and the sustained firing lasts only a few seconds. Therefore, it can be seen that upper motor neuron paralysis is characterized by rapidly firing MUAPs generating a complete interference pattern that is difficult to activate and poorly sustained.

The model of the motor unit is also helpful in understanding amplitude, duration, and phase changes in neuropathy and myopathy. It is useful to assume that the MUAP is the summation of potentials from several fibers in the same motor unit and that the fiber nearest the tip of the recording needle accounts for the major spike. Fibers further than 1 mm from the tip account for the low amplitude and slow initial and terminal phases of the motor unit potential, adding to its total duration.

In myopathy one can assume that some of the fibers in the motor unit are destroyed or nonfunctional, so one is less likely to record from distant fibers. Therefore, the initial and terminal forces are simply not there to be recorded, and the recorded motor unit potential is of shorter duration (less than 3 msec).

In neuropathy, after reinnervation of denervated muscle fibers by surviving motor neurons, more fibers are innervated by each surviving motor neuron. Therefore, a greater number of fibers in the same motor unit will be within "range" of the EMG needle and the total duration and amplitude of the single motor unit action potential may be increased (greater than 16 msec). For much the same reason amplitude is decreased in myopathy (fewer fibers per motor unit) and increased in neuropathy (more fibers per motor unit). Amplitude is so variable in normal MUAPs that only extremes of amplitude can be considered abnormal. Less than 300 μV is clearly a decrease and greater than 5 mV is definitely an increase.

The configuration of the MUAP loses its smooth diphasic, triphasic, or quadriphasic shape in both neuropathy and myopathy and becomes polyphasic (greater than four phases) (Fig. 18-19). The assumed explanations are somewhat different. In myopathy there is patchy loss of muscle fibers. The normal slight asynchrony of firing of the muscle fibers within a motor unit is accentuated, resulting in a polyphasic unit that is also of low amplitude and short duration. In neuropathy, the synchronous firing is interrupted by the incorporation of additional fibers into a motor unit. Neuropathic units are usually polyphasic if reinnervation has occurred, but end-stage units may simply be triphasic, of long duration, and of high amplitude. Because of the wide variation in amplitude and duration of normal MUAPs, those in mild degrees of myopathy and neuropathy may fall within the normal range.

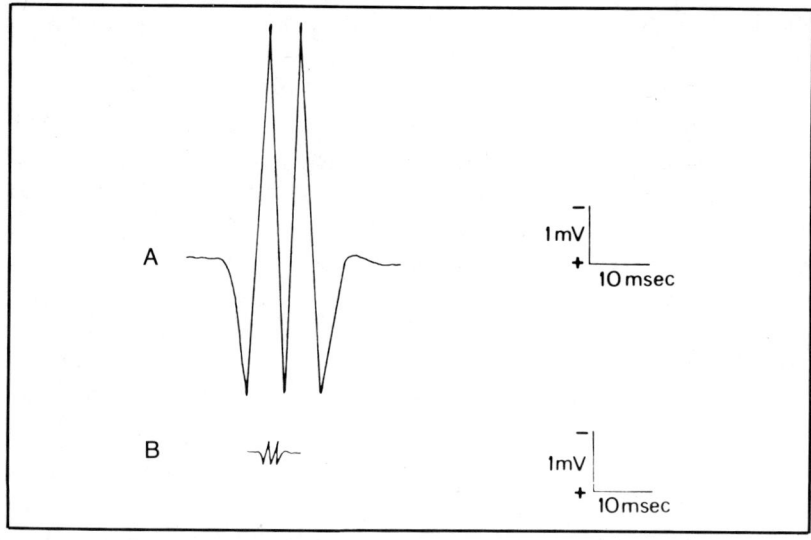

Figure 18-19
Neuropathic MUAP (A) and myopathic MUAP (B).

Table 18-8 summarizes the typical characteristics of MUAPs in myopathy, neuropathy, and normal muscle. Obviously there will be motor units with a mixture of these characteristics in every muscle examined. As previously discussed, different muscles tend to have different normal patterns of duration, amplitude, configuration, and recruitment. A great deal of experience is required to appreciate the enormous ranges of what is considered normal.

ANALYSIS OF ANATOMIC DISTRIBUTION

The question of abnormality in the EMG has three essential parts:

If? Normal versus abnormal
How? Myopathic versus neuropathic
Where? Generalized, proximal, distal, radicular, single nerve

A *myotome* is defined as a group of muscles supplied by a single spinal segment. The posterior primary ramus innervates the paraspinal muscles and the anterior primary ramus innervates the limb and girdle muscles (Fig. 18-20).

Table 18-8
Typical MUAP Characteristics in Myopathic, Neuropathic, and Normal Muscle

	Myopathy	Normal	Neuropathy
Duration	< 3 msec	3–16 msec	> 16 msec
Amplitude	< 300 μV	300 μV–5 mV	> 5 mV
Configuration	Polyphasic	Triphasic	Polyphasic

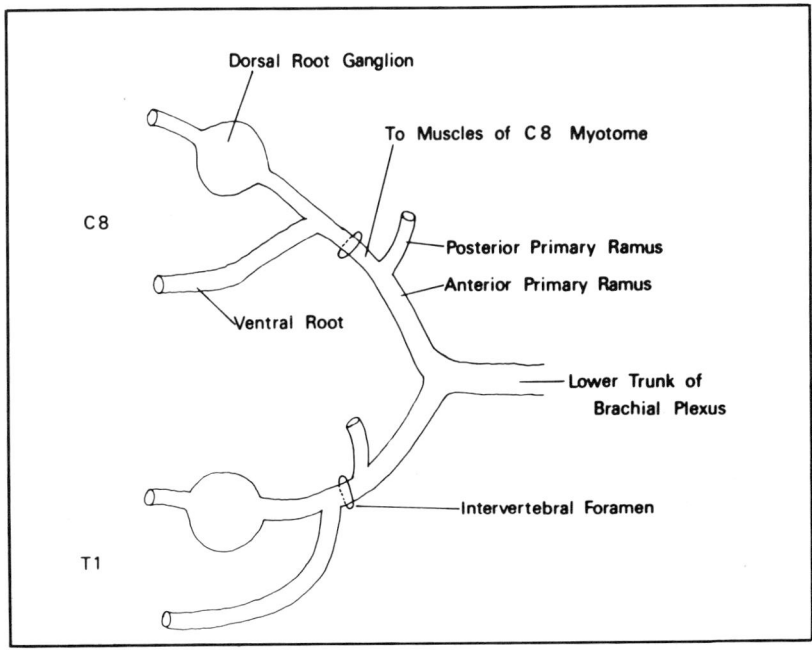

Figure 18-20
Anterior and posterior primary rami of a spinal nerve.

The innervation of paraspinous muscles such as the sacrospinalis muscle is diffusely overlapped. For instance, an abnormality detected in the sacrospinalis muscle between the fourth and fifth lumbar vertebrae may not be from the L_4 nerve root. The presence of abnormalities in the sacrospinalis muscle is helpful in differentiating a plexus (sacrospinalis not involved) from a root (sacrospinalis involved) lesion, but is not helpful in definite segmental localization. The deeper paraspinous muscles such as the multifidus are more selectively innervated by a single root, but their examination is technically demanding. Muscles often belong to more than one myotome. Most muscles are innervated by more than one spinal segment and are innervated in varying degrees by the different segments. For example, the tibialis anterior muscle receives its major innervation from L_4, but L_5 and S_1 contribute to a lesser degree. Unfortunately, there is also some disagreement about the root distribution to the various muscles. Therefore, the degree of abnormality, as well as the distribution of the abnormality, has to be considered. Table 18-9 lists the muscles and muscle groups which are reasonably accessible to needle study in actual practice.

The question of myotomal versus peripheral nerve involvement can usually be answered by the study of some or all of these muscles.

For the beginner it is useful to approach the question as follows:

1. Could the C_5 segment be involved?
2. Do the findings suggest that additional segments are involved?
3. Do the results definitely exclude the possibility of a single peripheral nerve lesion?

Table 18-10 lists the myotomes for cervical segments five, six, and seven [2, 3, 6, 10]. By reference to this table one can see that if the biceps is involved, the C_5 root *might* be involved, but the C_6 and C_7 roots *could* be involved as well. If the abnormalities are also present in the supraspinatus (C_5, C_6) and brachioradialis (C_5, C_6) but not in the deltoid (C_6, C_7) or flexor carpi ulnaris (C_7), it is probably C_5 rather than C_6. In practice, it is often possible only to localize the lesion to two adjacent segments (e.g., C_5 and C_6). The involvement of muscles innervated by different peripheral nerves excludes a single peripheral nerve lesion as the cause, but does not exclude plexus lesions. The readily accessible muscles are listed by myotome in Appendix VII. If one examines some of the various listings of myotomes available [2, 3, 6, 10], it will be

18. The EMG Examination

Table 18-9
Muscles Easily Accessible for EMG Study

Lower Extremity	Upper Extremity
Gluteus maximus	Trapezius
Gluteus medius/minimus	Supraspinatus
Adductors of thigh	Infraspinatus
Quadriceps femoris	Deltoid
Biceps femoris	Biceps
Tibialis anterior	Triceps
Gastrocnemius	Extensor digitorum communis
Soleus	Extensor carpi radialis longus
Peroneus longus/brevis	Flexor carpi ulnaris
Tibialis posterior	Pronator teres
Extensor digitorum brevis	Brachioradialis
Abductor digiti quinti	Opponens pollicis
	Abductor pollicis brevis
	Abductor digiti quinti
	First dorsal interosseous

Table 18-10
The Fifth, Sixth, and Seventh Cervical Myotomes

C_5	C_6	C_7
Supraspinatus	Biceps	Extensor carpi radialis longus
Infraspinatus	Brachioradialis	Pronator teres
Biceps	Extensor carpi radialis longus	Triceps
Deltoid	Pronator teres	Extensor digitorum
Brachioradialis	Supraspinatus	Deltoid
Extensor carpi radialis longus	Infraspinatus	Biceps
	Triceps	Flexor carpi ulnaris
	Deltoid	

noticed that they are not in complete agreement. This handbook emphasizes the more commonly accepted segmental innervations of the readily accessible muscles (Table 18-9) in order to start the beginner on the road to knowledge of segmental localization.

THE EMG REPORT

The EMG report should contain the findings in each muscle tested. Insertional activity and spontaneous activity are mentioned, and the characteristics of the motor unit action potentials are described. Amplitude, duration, and interference pattern (recruitment) are usually described as decreased, normal, or increased; polyphasia is commented upon if present to an abnormal degree. The EMG report should next summarize the electrophysiological findings to indicate the location of the lesion or lesions. This information should then be translated into a differential diagnosis. Appendix III contains an acceptable form for the EMG report.

REFERENCES

1. Buchthal, F., and Rosenfalck, P. Action potential parameters in different human muscles. *Acta Psychiatr. Neurol. Scand.* 30:125, 1955.
2. Goodgold, J., and Eberstein, A. *Electrodiagnosis of Neuromuscular Diseases* (2nd ed.). Baltimore: Williams & Wilkins, 1977.
3. Gross, C. M. (Ed.). *Gray's Anatomy* (29th American Edition). Philadelphia: Lea & Febiger, 1973.
4. Johnson, E. W. (Ed.). *Practical Electromyography*. Baltimore: Williams & Wilkins, 1980.
5. Licht, S. (Ed.). *Electrodiagnosis and Electromyography* (3rd ed.). New Haven: Licht, 1971.
6. Liveson, J. A., and Spielholz, N. I. *Peripheral Neurology*. Philadelphia: Davis, 1979.
7. Petajan, J. H., and Philip, B. A. Frequency control of motor unit action potentials. *Electroencephalogr. Clin. Neurophysiol.* 27:66, 1969.
8. Petajan, J. H. Clinical electromyographic studies of the diseases of the motor unit. *Electroencephalogr. Clin. Neurophysiol.* 36:395, 1974.
9. Petajan, J. H. Personal communication, 1980.
10. Riddoch, Brigadier G. (Chairman). *Aids to the Investigation of*

Peripheral Nerve Injuries (2nd ed.). London: Her Majesty's Stationery Office, 1943.
11. Sacco, G., Buchthal, F., and Rosenfalck, P. Motor unit potentials at different ages. *Arch. Neurol.* 6:44, 1962.
12. Walton, J. N. (Ed.). *Disorders of voluntary muscle* (3rd ed.). Edinburgh: Churchill Livingstone, 1974.

APPENDIXES

I Amplitudes of EMAPs Recorded from Selected Muscles (mV)

First dorsal interosseous	15 (6–22)
Abductor digiti quinti	11.3 (6–16)
Thenar muscles	11.8 (7–17)
Extensor muscles of forearm	10.5 (8–14)
Plantar muscles	15.4 (8–22)
Muscles of dorsum pedis	8.8 (6–12)

Source: Adapted from R. Hodes, M. G. Larrabee, and W. German. The human electromyogram in response to nerve stimulation and the conduction velocity of motor axons. *Arch. Neurol. Psychiatry* 60:340, 1948. Copyright 1948, American Medical Association. Used by permission.

II Durations of EMAPs Recorded by Stimulation of Selected Nerves (msec)

Median	15.7 ± 2.4 SD
Ulnar	14.0 ± 2.14 SD
Deep peroneal	14.9 ± 3.3 SD

Source: Adapted from B. G. B. Christie and E. N. Coomes. Normal variation of nerve conduction in three peripheral nerves. *Ann. Phys. Med.* 5:303, 1959–1960. Used by permission.

III The EMG Report Form

Muscle	Insertional Activity	Spontaneous Activity	MUAP

NCV Findings: _____

_____

Summary: _____

_____

Diagnosis: _____

_____

IV Normal Conduction Velocities and Distal Latencies

Nerve	Conduction Velocity (m/sec)	Distal Latency (msec)
Ulnar (Motor)		
Wrist to ADQ	...	2.8–4.2
Below elbow to wrist	45.2–55.3	...
Above elbow to wrist	45.2–55.3	...
Axilla to above elbow	44.9–60.6	...
Erb's point to axilla	55.0–73.2	...
Erb's point to above elbow	51.0–72.9	...
Ulnar (Sensory)		
Orthodromic	...	2.8 ± 0.2
Antidromic	...	3.2 ± 0.3
Median (Motor)		
Wrist to APB	...	3.4–4.5
Elbow to wrist	45.1–54.4	...
Axilla to elbow	50.0–68.3	...
Erb's to axilla	57.1–76.2	...
Erb's to elbow	51.0–76.0	...
Median (Sensory)		
Orthodromic	...	3.0 ± 0.25
Antidromic	...	3.2 ± 0.25
Radial (Motor)		
Forearm to EIP	...	2.4 ± 0.5
Elbow to forearm	62 ± 5.1	...
Axilla to elbow	69 ± 5.6	...
Erb's point to elbow	56–93	...

Nerve	Conduction Velocity (m/sec)	Distal Latency (msec)
Radial (Sensory)		
Antidromic	...	< 2.8
Musculocutaneous (Sensory)		
Antidromic	...	< 2.6
Sciatic (Motor)		
Gluteal fold to popliteal fossa	45.3–61.1	...
Peroneal (Motor)		
Ankle to EDB	...	5.1
Proximal to head of fibula to ankle	50 ± 3.5	...
Distal to head of fibula to ankle	50 ± 3.5	...
Superficial peroneal (Sensory)		
Antidromic	...	< 3.7
Posterior tibia (Motor)		
Above malleolus to AH	...	≤ 6.1
Above malleolus to ADQ	...	≤ 6.7
Popliteal fossa to above malleolus	43.4–59.5	...
Sural (Sensory)		
Antidromic	...	< 4.6
Femoral (Motor)		
Above inguinal ligament to VM	...	7.1
Below inguinal ligament to VM	...	6.0
Hunter's canal to VM	...	4.0
Above inguinal ligament to Hunter's canal	66.7	...
Below inguinal ligament to Hunter's canal	69.4	...
Saphenous (Sensory)		
Antidromic	...	3.6 ± 0.4

ADQ = Abductor digiti quinti
AH = Abductor hallucis
EDB = Extensor digitorum brevis
EIP = Extensor indicis proprius
VM = Vastus medialis

V. The Innervation of Commonly Studied Muscles by Named Nerves and Spinal Segments

Muscle	Nerve	Segment
Gluteus maximus	Inferior gluteal	$L_5; S_{1,2}$
Gluteus medius/minimus	Superior gluteal	$L_{4,5}; S_1$
Adductors of thigh	Obturator	$L_{2,3,4}$
Quadriceps femoris	Femoral	$L_{2,3,4}$
Biceps femoris	Sciatic trunk	$L_5; S_{1,2}$
Tibialis anterior	Deep peroneal	$L_{4,5}; S_1$
Gastrocnemius	Posterior tibial	$L_5; S_{1,2}$
Soleus	Posterior tibial	$L_5; S_{1,2}$
Peroneus longus/brevis	Superficial peroneal	$L_{4,5}; S_1$
Tibialis posterior	Posterior tibial	$L_{4,5}; S_1$
Extensor digitorum brevis	Deep peroneal	$L_{4,5}; S_1$
Abductor digiti quinti	Posterior tibial	$L_5; S_{1,2}$
Trapezius	Spinal accessory	$C_{3,4}$
Supraspinatus	Suprascapular	$C_{5,6}$
Infraspinatus	Suprascapular	$C_{5,6}$
Deltoid	Circumflex	$C_{3,4,5,6,7}$
Biceps	Musculocutaneous	$C_{5,6,7}$
Triceps	Radial	$C_{6,7,8}; T_1$
Extensor digitorum communis	Radial	$C_{7,8}$
Extensor carpi radialis longus	Radial	$C_{5,6,7,8}$
Flexor carpi ulnaris	Ulnar	$C_{7,8}; T_1$
Pronator teres	Median	$C_{6,7}$
Brachioradialis	Radial	$C_{5,6}$
Opponens pollicis	Median	$C_8; T_1$

Muscle	Nerve	Segment
Abductor pollicis brevis	Median	C_8; T_1
Abductor digiti quinti	Ulnar	C_8; T_1
First dorsal interosseous	Ulnar	C_8; T_1

VI The Major Motor Distributions of Commonly Studied Nerves

Nerve	Muscle(s)
Superior gluteal	Gluteus medius/minimus
Inferior gluteal	Gluteus maximus
Sciatic trunk	Biceps femoris
Superficial peroneal	Peroneus longus/brevis
Deep peroneal	Tibialis anterior
	Extensor digitorum brevis
Posterior tibial	Gastrocnemius
	Soleus
	Tibialis posterior
	Abductor digiti quinti
Obturator	Adductors of thigh
Femoral	Quadriceps femoris
Spinal accessory	Trapezius
Suprascapular	Supraspinatus
	Infraspinatus
Circumflex	Deltoid
Musculocutaneous	Biceps
Radial	Triceps
	Extensor digitorum communis
	Extensor carpi radialis longus
	Brachioradialis
Median	Pronator teres
	Opponens pollicis
	Abductor pollicis brevis
Ulnar	Flexor carpi ulnaris
	Abductor digiti quinti
	First dorsal interosseous

VII Myotomes of the Upper and Lower Extremities

L_2 *Myotome*
Adductors of thigh
Quadriceps femoris

L_3 *Myotome*
Adductors of thigh
Quadriceps femoris

L_4 *Myotome*
Gluteus medius/minimus
Adductors of thigh
Quadriceps femoris
Tibialis anterior
Peroneus longus/brevis
Tibialis posterior
Extensor digitorum brevis

L_5 *Myotome*
Gluteus maximus
Gluteus medius/minimus
Biceps femoris
Tibialis anterior
Gastrocnemius
Peroneus longus/brevis
Tibialis posterior
Extensor digitorum brevis
Abductor digiti quinti

S_1 *Myotome*
Gluteus maximus
Gluteus medius/minimus
Biceps femoris
Tibialis anterior
Gastrocnemius
Soleus
Peroneus longus/brevis
Tibialis posterior
Extensor digitorum brevis
Abductor digiti quinti

S_2 *Myotome*
Gluteus maximus
Biceps femoris
Gastrocnemius
Soleus
Abductor digiti quinti

C_3 *Myotome*
Trapezius
Deltoid

C_4 *Myotome*
Trapezius
Deltoid

C_5 *Myotome*
Supraspinatus
Infraspinatus

Deltoid
Biceps
Extensor carpi radialis longus
Brachioradialis

C_6 Myotome
Supraspinatus
Infraspinatus
Deltoid
Biceps
Triceps
Extensor carpi radialis longus
Pronator teres
Brachioradialis

C_7 Myotome
Deltoid
Biceps
Triceps
Extensor digitorum communis

Extensor carpi radialis longus
Flexor carpi ulnaris
Pronator teres

C_8 Myotome
Triceps
Extensor digitorum communis
Extensor carpi radialis longus
Flexor carpi ulnaris
Opponens pollicis
Abductor pollicis brevis
Abductor digiti quinti
First dorsal interosseous

T_1 Myotome
Triceps
Flexor carpi ulnaris
Opponens pollicis
Abductor pollicis brevis
Abductor digiti quinti
First dorsal interosseous

VIII The EMG Examination: Characteristics of Spontaneous and Exertional Activity

Characteristics	Fibrillations	Positive Sharp Waves	Fasciculations
Amplitude	20–300 μV	120 ± 45 μV Rarely up to 4 mV	300 μV–5 mV
Duration	1–5 msec	10–100 msec	3–16 msec
Frequency	1–30 per second	10/sec Range 2–100	1–50 per *minute*
Firing Interval	Regular	Variable, usually regular	Irregular
Configuration	Diphasic, triphasic; initial deflection positive	Diphasic; abrupt, initial positive deflection	Diphasic to polyphasic; initial deflection positive
Sound	Rain on the roof or high pitched clicks	Dull, popping	Dull pop

Characteristics	MEPP	"Nerve" Potential	Normal MUAP
Amplitude	10–100 μV	10–200 μV	300 μV–5 mV
Duration	1–2 msec	3–5 msec	3–16 msec
Frequency	20–25 per second	up to 50/sec	Variable 5–50 per second
Firing Interval	Irregular	Irregular	Regular
Configuration	Diphasic; initial deflection negative	Diphasic; initial deflection negative	Diphasic, triphasic, quadriphasic; initial deflection positive
Sound	Seashell held to ear	Buzzing, crackling	Sharp, crisp pop when motor unit near needle tip

IX Motor Points of Commonly Studied Muscles

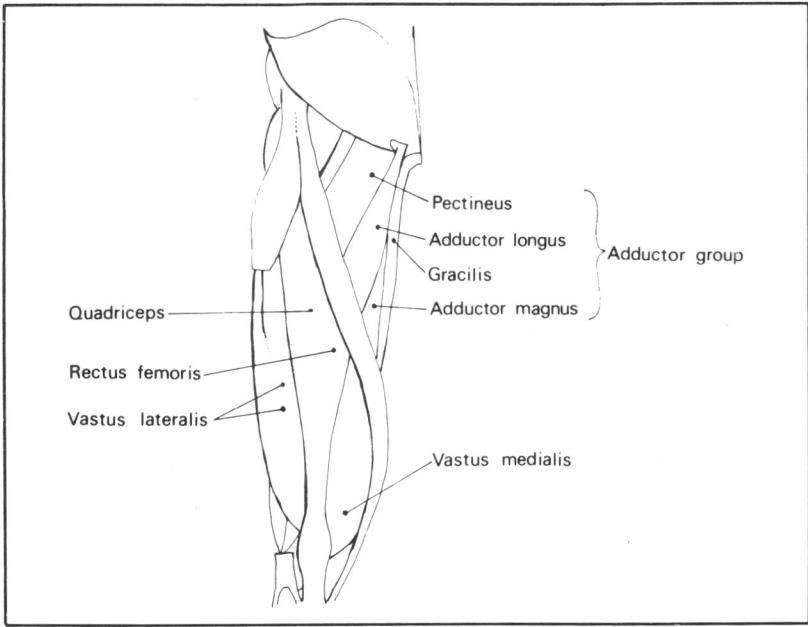

The anterior thigh.

Illustrations redrawn from S. Licht (Ed.). *Electrodiagnosis and Electromyography* (3rd ed.). New Haven: Licht, 1971.

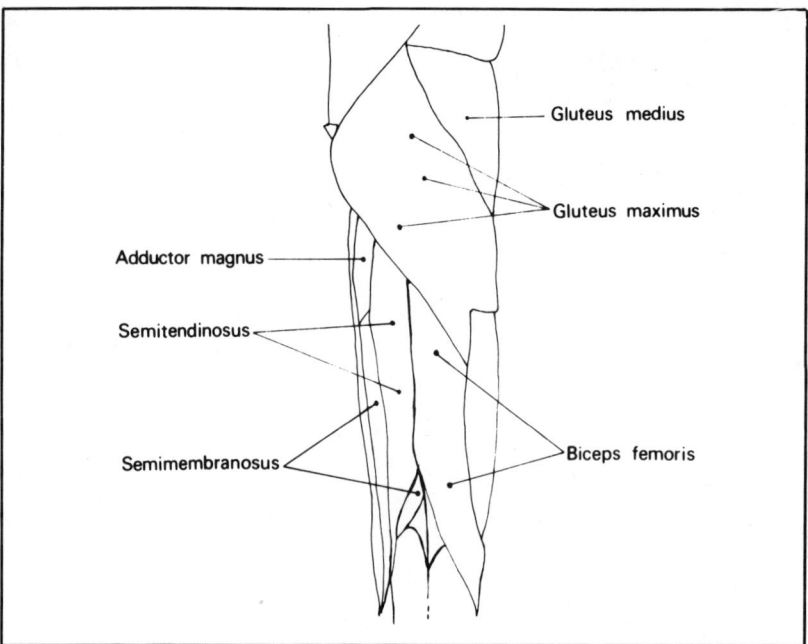

The posterior thigh.

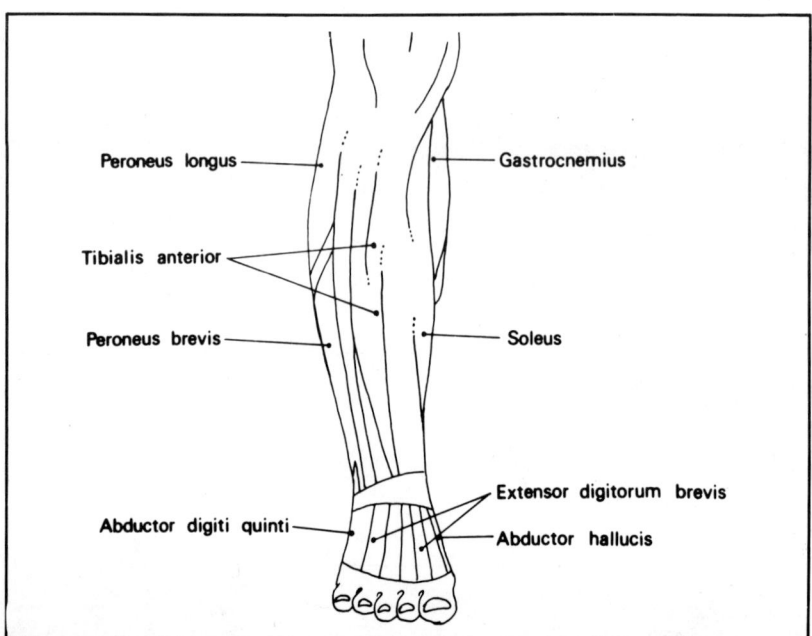

The anterior leg.

145 *Appendixes*

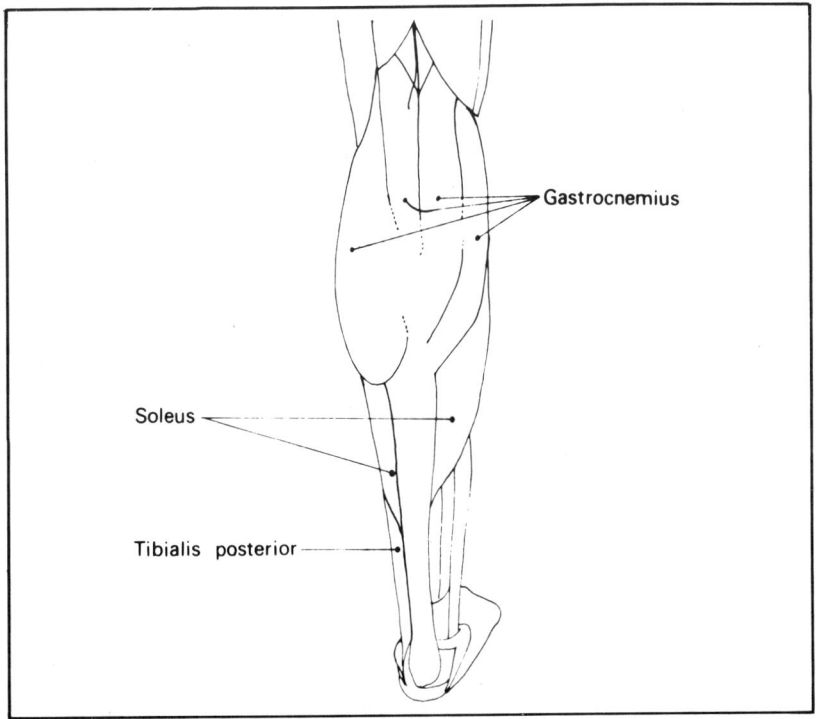

The posterior leg.

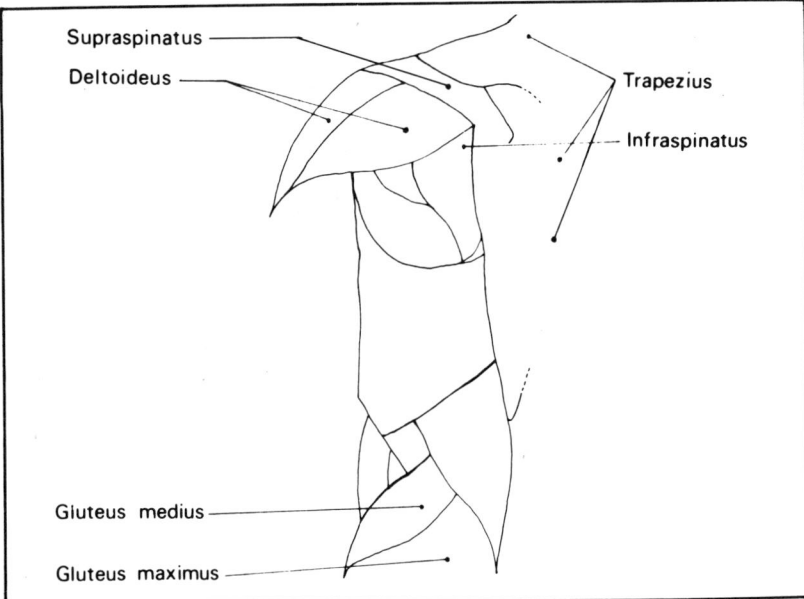

The posterior trunk.

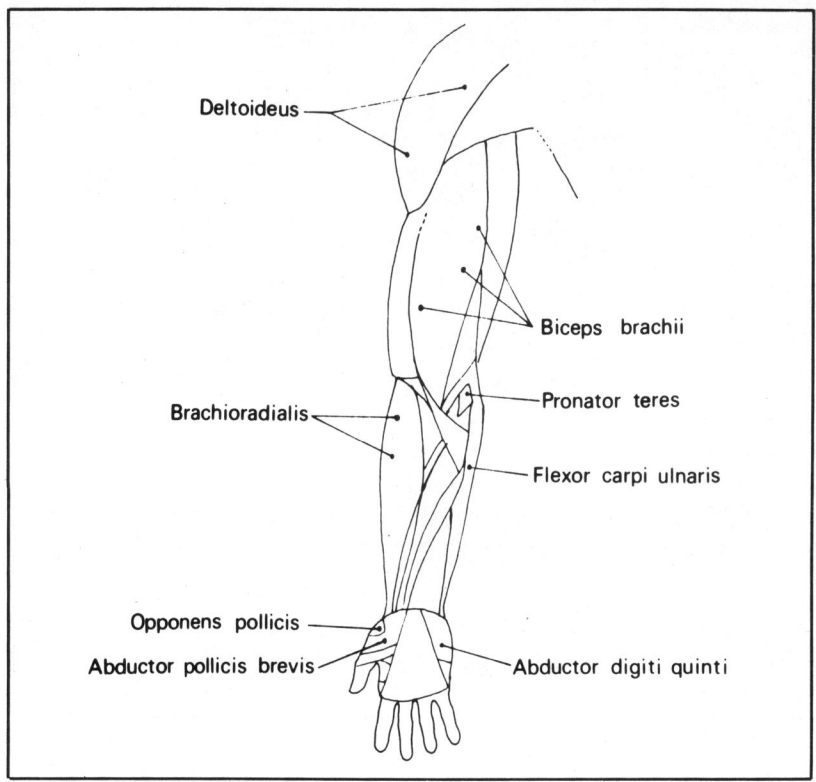

The anterior upper extremity.

147 *Appendixes*

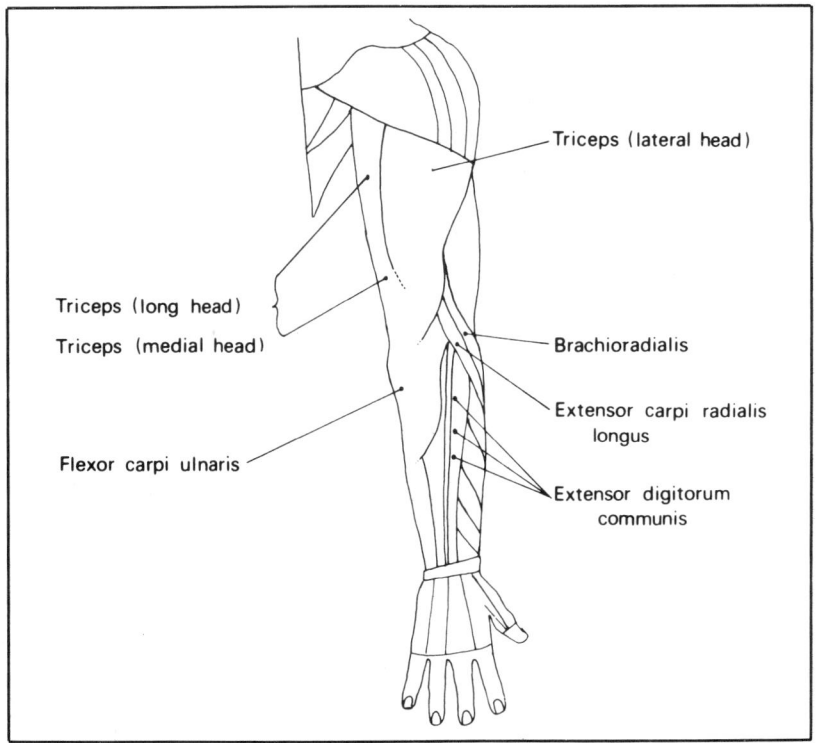

The posterior upper extremity.

INDEX

Index

Abductor digiti quinti
  accessible for EMG study, 125
  electrode placement for recording from, 50
  evoked muscle action potential of, 131
  innervation of, 136, 137
  motor points for, 144, 146
  motor unit action potential for, 113, 115
Abductor hallucis
  electrode placement for recording from, 63–64
  motor points for, 144
Abductor pollicis brevis
  accessible for EMG study, 125
  evoked muscle action potential from, 2
  innervation of, 137
  motor points for, 146
Adductor longus, motor points for, 143
Adductor magnus, motor points for, 143, 144
Adductors of thigh
  accessible for EMG study, 125
  innervation of, 136
Age, and motor nerve conduction velocities, 10
Alcoholism
  contracture associated with, 108
  femoral nerve in, 71
Alkalosis, cramp associated with, 108
Amplitude, recording, 9
Anterior horn cell disease, proximal shoulder girdle muscles in, 13
Anterior interosseous syndrome, median nerve in, 27
Antidromic stimulation, 5
Axilla, as stimulation point, 5, 9

Bell's palsy, 81
Biceps brachi
  accessible for EMG study, 125
  and cervical myotomes, 125
  electrode placement for, 15
  innervation of, 136
  motor points for, 146
  motor unit action potential for, 113, 115
  onset and recruitment intervals in, 119
  polyphasic potentials in, 114
Biceps femoris
  accessible for EMG study, 125
  innervation of, 136
  motor points for, 144
  motor unit action potential
  onset and recruitment intervals in, 119
  polyphasic potentials in, 114
Brachial plexus, 12, 13
  nerve conduction procedure for, 14–17
  normal mean latencies for, 14
  stimulation site for, 14
Brachial plexus neuritis, proximal shoulder girdle muscles in, 13
Brachioradialis
  accessible for EMG study, 125
  and cervical myotomes, 125
  innervation of, 136
  motor points for, 146, 147
  onset and recruitment intervals in, 119

Cervical disc herniation, proximal shoulder girdle muscles in, 13
Circumflex nerve, motor distribution of, 138
Conduction velocities
  calculation of, 1–2
  normal, 134–135

Configuration, recording, 9
Continuous muscle fiber activity syndrome, 108–109
Cramp
  characteristics of, 108
  myokymia associated with, 107
Cranial nerve, seventh, anatomy of, 81

Deltoid
  accessible for EMG study, 125
  and cervical myotomes, 125
  electrode placement for, 15
  innervation of, 136
  motor points for, 145, 146
  motor unit action potential in, 113
  onset and recruitment intervals in, 119
Diabetes mellitus, femoral nerve in, 71
Discharges
  complex repetitive, 105
  grouped motor unit, 107
Distal latencies, normal, 134–135
Dorsal cutaneous nerves, 59. *See also* Musculocutaneous nerve (forearm)
Dorsum pedis, evoked muscle action potential of muscles of, 131
Drugs, cramp associated with, 108

Electrodes
  concentric, 100, 101
  monopolar, 100, 101, 102
  recording, 5, 6
  stimulating, 4, 7
  types of, 6–7
EMAP. *See* Evoked muscle action potential (EMAP)
Erb's point
  anatomic location of, 5
  stimulation of, 8
Evoked muscle action potential (EMAP), 2
  from abductor pollicis brevis, 2
  duration of, 132
  recording, 3
  of vastus medialis, 71
Evoked sensory action potential, from median nerve, 4
Examination, EMG
  exertional activity in, 110
  insertional activity in, 102–103
  spontaneous activity in, 103–109
Exertional activity
  characteristics of, 141–142
  in EMG exam, 110–122
Extensor carpi radialis longus
  accessible for EMG study, 125
  and cervical myotomes, 125
  innervation of, 136
  motor points for, 147
Extensor digitorum brevis (foot)
  accessible for EMG study, 125
  innervation of, 136
  motor points for, 144
  motor unit action potential in, 113
  onset and recruitment intervals in, 119
  polyphasic potentials in, 114
Extensor digitorum communis (forearm)
  accessible for EMG study, 125
  evoked muscle action potential of, 131
  innervation of, 136
  motor points for, 147
  seventh cervical myotome, 125
Extensor indicis proprius, electrode placement for recording from, 36

Facial muscles
  onset and recruitment intervals in, 119
  polyphasic potentials in, 114
Facial nerve
  electrode placement for, 82–83
  and mastoid process of temporal bone, 80
  normal motor values for, 83
  stimulation of, 84
Fasciculations, 106–107
Femoral nerve
  anatomy of, 71, 77
  conduction velocity for, 135
  distal latency for, 135
  motor distribution of, 138
  normal motor values, 75
  origin and course of, 70
  stimulation of, 72, 73, 74
Fibrillation potentials
  essential characteristics of, 104
  recording of, 103–104
Flexor carpi ulnaris
  accessible for EMG study, 125
  innervation of, 136
  motor points for, 146, 147
  and seventh cervical myotome, 125
F-waves
  anatomy and physiology of, 87
  electrode placement for, 88
  normal parameters of, 87
  normal values for, 89
  variation of latency, amplitude, and configuration in, 86

Gastrocnemius
  accessible for EMG study, 125

innervation of, 136
motor points for, 144, 145
motor unit action potential in, 113
onset and recruitment intervals in, 119
polyphasic potentials in, 114
Gluteal nerves, motor distribution of, 138
Gluteus maximus
accessible for EMG study, 125
innervation of, 136
motor points for, 144, 145
onset and recruitment intervals in, 119
Gluteus medius
accessible for EMG study, 125
innervation of, 136
motor points for, 144, 145
Gracilis, motor points of, 143
Ground, for ulnar nerve stimulation, 20
Grouped motor unit discharges, 107
Guillain-Barré syndrome, F-wave latencies in, 88

Handcuff neuropathy, radial nerve in, 35
H-reflex
anatomy and physiology of, 91
applications of, 91–92
electrode placement for, 93
eliciting, 90
normal latency values for, 94
procedure for, 92
Hunter's canal, stimulation point at, 74
Hyperhidrosis, myokymia in, 107
Hypocalcemia, cramp associated with, 108
Hypokalemia, contracture associated with, 108

Infraspinatus
accessible for EMG study, 125
and cervical myotomes, 125
electrode placement for, 17
innervation of, 136
motor points for, 145
Insertional activity, 102–103
Interference patterns, 116, 117
Interosseous, first dorsal
accessible for EMG study, 125
evoked muscle action potential of, 131
innervation of, 137
onset and recruitment intervals in, 119

Lambert-Eaton syndrome, Evoked muscle action potential in, 95, 97
Latency
definition of, 1
with F-waves, 87
measurements of, 3, 13
motor, 2–3
normal distal, 134–135

Ligament of Struther's syndrome, median nerve in, 27
Lumbosacral plexus
anatomy of, 47, 77
simplified plan of, 46

McArdle's disease, contracture associated with, 108
Median nerve
anatomy of, 27
antidromic procedure for, 30
conduction velocities for, 134
distal latencies for, 134
electrode placement for, 29, 30, 31
evoked muscle action potential of, 132
evoked sensory action potential (ESAP) of, 4
motor distribution of, 138
normal motor values, 28
normal sensory values, 30, 31
origin and course of, 26
orthodromic procedure, 28
stimulation of, 29
Miniature end-plate potentials (MEPP), 109, 110
Motor nerve, repetitive supramaximal stimulation of, 95
Motor unit, exertional activity of, 120
Motor unit action potential (MUAP), 101
amplitude of, 115
configuration of, 115
duration of, 111, 113, 115
essential characteristics of, 111
normal, 110
single, 112
M-response, in H-reflex, 91
MUAP. See Motor unit action potential (MUAP)
Muscles
accessible for EMG study, 125
evoked muscle action potential from, 131
innervation of, 136
motor points of, 143
Muscular atrophy, myokymia in, 107
Musculocutaneous nerve (forearm)
anatomy of, 43
antidromic procedure for, 43
conduction velocity for, 135
distal latency for, 135
electrode placement for, 44
motor distribution of, 138
normal sensory values for, 44
superficial course of, 42
Myasthenia gravis, evoked muscle action potential in, 95, 97–98

Myasthenic syndromes, proximal shoulder girdle muscles in, 13
Myokymia, 107
Myoneural relationship, measurements of, 102
Myopathy
  motor unit action potential in, 121, 122, 123
  onset and recruitment intervals in, 119
Myotomes
  cervical, 125
  definition of, 122
  identification of, 139–140
Myotonia, electrical, 106

NCV (Nerve conduction velocity), calculation of, 1–2
"Needle" examination, 101
Nerve conduction studies
  motor, 2–3
  sensory, 3
Nerve conduction velocity (NCV), calculation of, 1–2
Nerve entrapment syndromes, proximal shoulder girdle muscles in, 13
"Nerve" potentials, 109–110. *See also* Evoked muscle action potential (EMAP); Motor unit action potential (MUAP)
Nerves, major motor distributions of, 138
Neuromyotonia, 108–109
Neuropathies
  fasciculations in, 106
  F-wave latencies in, 88
  handcuff, 35
  motor unit action potential in, 121, 122, 123
  onset and recruitment intervals in, 119

Obturator nerve, motor distribution of, 138
Opponens pollicis
  accessible for EMG study, 125
  innervation of, 136
  motor points for, 146
  motor unit action potential in, 113
Orthodromic stimulation, 5

Paralysis, upper motor neuron, 120–121
Paresthesias, peroneal nerve in, 53
Pectineus, motor points of, 143
Peroneal nerve
  conduction velocity for, 135
  distal latency for, 135
Peroneal nerve, common, 47
  anatomy of, 53
  electrode placement for, 54, 55

motor branches, 52
normal motor values, 56
stimulation of, 54, 55
Peroneal nerve, deep
  evoked muscle action potential of, 132
  motor distribution of, 138
Peroneal nerve, superficial
  anatomy of, 59
  antidromic procedure for, 59–60
  distal sensory branches, 58
  electrode placement for, 60
  motor distribution of, 138
  normal sensory values, 60
Peroneus longus, motor unit action potential in, 113
Peroneus longus brevis
  accessible for EMG study, 125
  innervation of, 136
  motor points for, 144
Phosphofructokinase deficiency, contracture associated with, 108
Plantar muscles, evoked muscle action potential of, 131
Plantar nerve, lateral, anatomy of, 63
Polyneuritis, proximal shoulder girdle muscles in, 13
Polyneuropathies. *See also* Neuropathies
  musculocutaneous nerve in, 43
  superficial peroneal nerve in, 59
  sural nerve in, 67
Polyphasia, degree of, 112
Popliteal aneurysm, tibial nerve in, 63
Posterior interosseous syndrome, radial nerve in, 35
Pronator syndrome, median nerve in, 27
Pronator teres
  accessible for EMG study, 125
  and cervical myotomes, 125
  innervation of, 136
  motor points for, 146
  onset and recruitment intervals in, 119

Quadriceps femoris
  accessible for EMG study, 125
  innervation of, 136
  motor points of, 143

Radial nerve
  motor
    anatomy of, 35
    antidromic procedure for, 37, 39
    conduction velocities for, 134
    distal latencies for, 134
    electrode placement for stimulation of, 36
    motor distribution of, 138

normal motor values for, 37, 39
  origin and course of, 34
  stimulation of, 37
sensory
  normal values for, 39
  superficial course of, 38
Radiculopathies
  saphenous nerve in, 77
  sural nerve in, 67
Recruitment interval, 114
Rectus femoris, motor points of, 143
Report, EMG, 9, 126, 133
Rheumatoid arthritis, F-wave latencies in, 88

Saphenous nerve, 71
  anatomy of, 77
  antidromic procedure for, 77
  conduction velocity for, 135
  distal latency for, 135
  distal superficial course of, 76
  electrode placement for, 77–78
  normal sensory values, 78
  stimulation of, 77–78
"Saturday night" palsies, radial nerve in, 35
Sciatic nerve, 47
  conduction velocity for, 135
  distal latency for, 135
  electrode placement for, 49
  locating superficial portion of, 48
  motor distribution of, 138
  posterior tibial branch of, 51
  stimulation of, 49, 50, 51
  "Sciatic" palsy, 49
Semimembranosus, motor points for, 144
Semitendinosus, motor points for, 144
Sodium depletion, cramp associated with, 108
Soleus
  accessible for EMG study, 125
  innervation of, 136
  motor points for, 144, 145
Spinal accessory nerve, motor distribution of, 138
Spinal nerves
  anatomy of, 47
  rami of, 123
Spontaneous activity
  abnormal, 103–109
  characteristics of, 141–142
  complex repetitive discharges, 105
  contracture, 108
  cramp, 108
  electrical myotonia, 106–107
  fasciculations, 106–107

fibrillations, 103–104
  myokymia, 107
  neuromyotonia, 108–109
  normal, 109–110
  positive sharp waves, 104–105
  stiff-man syndrome, 108
Stiff-man syndrome, 108
Stimulation of nerves
  antidromic, 5
  orthodromic, 5
  repetitive supramaximal, 95–98
Stimulation points, 5
Stylomastoid foramen
  and facial nerve stimulation, 83
  and mastoid process of temporal bone, 80
Suprascapular nerve, motor distribution of, 138
Supraspinatus
  accessible for EMG study, 125
  and cervical myotomes, 125
  electrode placement, 16
  innervation of, 136
  motor points for, 145
Sural nerve
  anatomy of, 67
  antidromic procedure for, 67, 69
  conduction velocity for, 135
  distal latency for, 135
  electrode placement for, 68
  normal sensory values, 69
  origin and course of, 66
  stimulation of, 68

Tarsal tunnel syndrome, tibial nerve in, 63
Tennis elbow, radial nerve in, 35
Tetany, myokymia in, 107
Thenar muscles, evoked muscle action potential of, 131
Thyrotoxicosis
  fasciculations in, 106
  myokymia in, 107
Tibial nerve, posterior, 47
  anatomy of, 53, 63
  conduction velocity for, 135
  distal latency for, 135
  electrode placement for, 63–64
  and H-reflex, 90
  motor distribution of, 138
  normal motor values, 65
  origin and course of, 62
  stimulation of, 93
Tibialis anterior
  accessible for EMG study, 125
  innervation of, 124, 136
  motor points for, 144

Tibialis anterior—*Continued*
    motor unit action potential in, 113
    onset and recruitment intervals in, 119
    polyphasic potentials in, 114
Tibialis posterior
    accessible for EMG study, 125
    innervation of, 136
    motor points for, 145
Trapezius
    accessible for EMG study, 125
    and cervical myotomes, 125
    innervation of, 136
    motor points for, 145
Triceps brachii
    accessible for EMG study, 125
    electrode placement for stimulation of, 16
    innervation of, 136
    motor points for, 147
    motor unit action potential in, 113
    onset and recruitment intervals in, 119

Ulnar nerve
    anatomy of, 19
    antidromic procedure, 23
    conduction velocities for, 134
    distal latencies for, 134
    electrode placement, 20–21, 23, 24
    evoked muscle action potential of, 132
    motor distribution of, 138
    normal motor values, 22
    normal sensory values, 22
    origin and course of, 18
    orthodromic procedure, 22
    stimulation of, 21
Uremia
    cramp associated with, 108
    myokymia associated with, 107

Vastus lateralis
    motor points of, 143
    onset and recruitment intervals in, 119
Vastus medialis
    electrode placement for recording from, 74
    evoked muscle action potentials from, 72
    motor points for, 143
Ventral ramus, of spinal nerves, 13

Waves, positive sharp, 104–105. *See also* F-waves